LEARNING GUIDE
WITH INTEGRATED REVIEW

INTRODUCTORY ALGEBRA
FOR COLLEGE STUDENTS
SEVENTH EDITION

P9-CDC-221

Robert Blitzer

Miami Dade College

PEARSON

Boston   Columbus   Indianapolis   New York   San Francisco
Amsterdam   Cape Town   Dubai   London   Madrid   Milan   Munich   Paris   Montreal   Toronto
Delhi   Mexico City   São Paulo   Sydney   Hong Kong   Seoul   Singapore   Taipei   Tokyo

The author and publisher of this book have used their best efforts in preparing this book. These efforts include the development, research, and testing of the theories and programs to determine their effectiveness. The author and publisher make no warranty of any kind, expressed or implied, with regard to these programs or the documentation contained in this book. The author and publisher shall not be liable in any event for incidental or consequential damages in connection with, or arising out of, the furnishing, performance, or use of these programs.

Reproduced by Pearson from electronic files supplied by the author.

Copyright © 2017, 2013, 2009 Pearson Education, Inc.
Publishing as Pearson, 501 Boylston Street, Boston, MA 02116.

All rights reserved. No part of this publication may be reproduced, stored in a retrieval system, or transmitted, in any form or by any means, electronic, mechanical, photocopying, recording, or otherwise, without the prior written permission of the publisher. Printed in the United States of America.

ISBN-13: 978-0-13-453950-8
ISBN-10: 0-13-453950-8

1 16

www.pearsonhighered.com

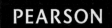

Introductory Algebra for College Students with Integrated Review 7e

Table of Contents

Section 1.1
Introduction to Algebra: Variables and Mathematical Models

Where Goes the Bride????

American's attitudes about marriage are changing.
More and more people are saying that marriage is optional and obsolete.

In this section of your textbook we explore how mathematics can be used to see how these attitudes vary by age group.

First Steps:

☐ **Take comprehensive notes** from your instructor's lecture and insert your notes into this section of the *Learning Guide*. Be sure to write down all examples, definitions, and other key concepts. Additional learning resources include the *Video Lecture Series*, the *PowerPoints*, and Section 1.1 of your textbook which begins on page 2.

☐ Complete the *Concept and Vocabulary Check* on page 10 of the textbook.

Guided Practice:

☐ Review each of the following *Solved Problems* and complete each *Pencil Problem*.

Learning Objective #1: Evaluate algebraic expressions.	
✔ *Solved Problem #1*	✎ *Pencil Problem #1* ✎
1a. Evaluate the expression $2(x+6)$ for $x=10$. $$2(x+6) = 2(\overset{x}{10}+6)$$ $$= 2(16)$$ $$= 32$$	**1a.** Evaluate the expression $5+3x$ for $x=4$.
1b. Evaluate the expression $\dfrac{6x-y}{2y-x-8}$ for $x=3$ and $y=8$. $$\dfrac{6x-y}{2y-x-8} = \dfrac{6\cdot\overset{x}{3}-\overset{y}{8}}{2\cdot\underset{y}{8}-\underset{x}{3}-8}$$ $$= \dfrac{18-8}{16-3-8}$$ $$= \dfrac{10}{5}$$ $$= 2$$	**1b.** Evaluate the expression $\dfrac{2x-y+6}{2y-x}$ for $x=7$ and $y=5$.

Copyright © 2017 Pearson Education, Inc.

Learning Objective #2: Translate English phrases into algebraic expressions.

✔ Solved Problem #2

2. Write each English phrase as an algebraic expression. Let the variable *x* represent the number.

2a. the product of 6 and a number

$6x$

2b. a number added to 4

$4 + x$

2c. three times a number, increased by 5

$3x + 5$

2d. twice a number subtracted from 12

$12 - 2x$

2e. the quotient of 15 and a number

$\dfrac{15}{x}$

✎ Pencil Problem #2✎

2. Write each English phrase as an algebraic expression. Let the variable *x* represent the number.

2a. four more than a number

2b. nine subtracted from a number

2c. three times a number, decreased by 5

2d. one less than the product of 12 and a number

2e. six more than the quotient of a number and 30

Learning Objective #3: Determine whether a number is a solution of an equation.

✔ Solved Problem #3

3a. Determine whether the given number is a solution of the equation.
$9x - 3 = 42; \ 6$

$9x - 3 = 42$
$9(6) - 3 = 42$
$54 - 3 = 42$
$\quad 51 = 42, \ \text{false}$

6 is not a solution.

3b. Determine whether the given number is a solution of the equation.
$2(y + 3) = 5y - 3; \ 3$

$2(y + 3) = 5y - 3$
$2(3 + 3) = 5(3) - 3$
$\quad 2(6) = 15 - 3$
$\quad\ 12 = 12, \ \text{true}$

3 is a solution.

✎ Pencil Problem #3✎

3a. Determine whether the given number is a solution of the equation.
$5a - 4 = 2a + 5; \ 3$

3b. Determine whether the given number is a solution of the equation.
$2(w + 1) = 3(w - 1); \ 7$

Copyright © 2017 Pearson Education, Inc.

Learning Objective #4: Translate English sentences into algebraic equations.

✔ *Solved Problem #4*

4a. Write the sentence as an equation. Let the variable x represent the number.

The quotient of a number and 6 is 5.

$$\frac{x}{6} = 5$$

4b. Write the sentence as an equation. Let the variable x represent the number.

Seven decreased by twice a number yields 1.

$7 - 2x = 1$

✎ *Pencil Problem #4*

4a. Write the sentence as an equation. Let the variable x represent the number.

Four times a number is 28.

4b. Write the sentence as an equation. Let the variable x represent the number.

Five times a number is equal to 24 decreased by the number.

Learning Objective #5: Evaluate formulas.

✔ *Solved Problem #5*

5. Divorce rates are considerably higher for couples who marry in their teens. The line graphs in the figure show the percentages of marriages ending in divorce based on the wife's age at marriage.

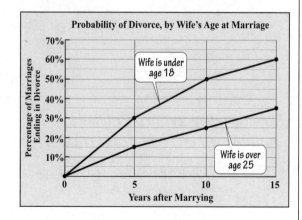

The following mathematical models approximate the data displayed by the line graphs.

Wife is under 18 at time of marriage:
$$d = 4n + 5$$

Wife is over 25 at time of marriage:
$$d = 2.3n + 1.5$$

✎ *Pencil Problem #5*

5. A bowler's handicap, H, is often found by using the following formula:

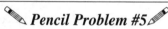
$$H = 0.8(200 - A)$$

where H represents the bowler's handicap and A is the bowler's average.

A bowler's final score for a game is the score for that game increased by the handicap.

5a. If your average bowling score is 145, what is your handicap?

Copyright © 2017 Pearson Education, Inc.

5a. Use the appropriate formula to determine the percentage of marriages ending in divorce after 15 years when the wife is under 18 at the time of marriage.

$d = 4n + 5$

$d = 4(15) + 5 = 65$

65% of marriages end in divorce after 15 years when the wife is under 18 at the time of marriage

5b. Use the appropriate line graph in the figure to determine the percentage of marriages ending in divorce after 15 years when the wife is under 18 at the time of marriage.

According to the line graph, 60% of marriages end in divorce after 15 years when the wife is under 18 at the time of marriage.

5c. Does the value given by the mathematical model underestimate or overestimate the actual percentage of marriages ending in divorce after 15 years as shown by the graph? By how much?

$65\% - 60\% = 5\%$

The mathematical model overestimates the actual percentage shown in the graph by 5%.

5b. What would your final score be if you bowled 120 in a game?

Answers for Pencil Problems *(Textbook Exercise references in parentheses)*:

1a. 17 *(1.1 #9)*   **1b.** 5 *(1.1 #23)*   **2a.** $x + 4$ *(1.1 #25)*   **2b.** $x - 9$ *(1.1 #31)*   **2c.** $3x - 5$ *(1.1 #35)*

2d. $12x - 1$ *(1.1 #37)*   **2e.** $\dfrac{x}{30} + 6$ *(1.1 #41)*   **3a.** solution *(1.1 #53)*   **3b.** not a solution *(1.1 #57)*

4a. $4x = 28$ *(1.1 #59)*   **4b.** $5x = 24 - x$ *(1.1 #73)*

5a. 44 *(1.1 #87a)*   **5b.** 164 *(1.1 #87b)*

Homework:

☐ **Review the Section 1.1 summary** that begins on page 102 of the textbook.

☐ **Insert your homework** into this section of the *Learning Guide*. Show all work neatly and check your answers. Strive to work through difficulties when possible, making note of any exercises where you need additional help. Remember, even if your instructor assigns homework through *MyMathLab*, you should still write out your work.

          Copyright © 2017 Pearson Education, Inc.

Section 1.2
Fractions in Algebra

> # What is Your Goal When You Exercise?
>
> Are you looking to boost your performance, lose weight, improve your overall health and reduce your risk of heart attack?
>
> Your target heart rate during exercise will differ depending on the specific goals you have.
>
> While completing the application exercises in this section of your textbook, you will utilize formulas to analyze the lower and upper limits of your target heart rate range.

First Steps:

☐ **Take comprehensive notes** from your instructor's lecture and insert your notes into this section of the *Learning Guide*. Be sure to write down all examples, definitions, and other key concepts. Additional learning resources include the *Video Lecture Series*, the *PowerPoints*, and Section 1.2 of your textbook which begins on page 14.

☐ Complete the *Concept and Vocabulary Check* on page 28 of the textbook.

Guided Practice:

☐ Review each of the following *Solved Problems* and complete each *Pencil Problem*.

Learning Objective #1: Convert between mixed numbers and improper fractions.	
✔ *Solved Problem #1*	✏ *Pencil Problem #1* ✏
1a. Convert $2\frac{5}{8}$ to an improper fraction.	**1a.** Convert $7\frac{3}{5}$ to an improper fraction.
$2\frac{5}{8} = \frac{2 \cdot 8 + 5}{8}$ $= \frac{16 + 5}{8}$ $= \frac{21}{8}$	
1b. Convert $\frac{5}{3}$ to a mixed number. 5 divided by 3 is 1 with a remainder of 2, so $\frac{5}{3} = 1\frac{2}{3}$.	**1b.** Convert $\frac{76}{9}$ to a mixed number.

Learning Objective #2: Write the prime factorization of a composite number.

✔ *Solved Problem #2*

2. Find the prime factorization of 36.

Begin by selecting any two numbers whose product is 36.
Here is one possibility: $36 = 4 \cdot 9$

Because the factors 4 and 9 are not prime, factor each of these composite numbers.
$36 = 4 \cdot 9$
$\quad = 2 \cdot 2 \cdot 3 \cdot 3$
Notice that 2 and 3 are both prime.

The prime factorization of 36 is $2 \cdot 2 \cdot 3 \cdot 3$.

✎ *Pencil Problem #2* ✎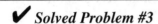

2. Find the prime factorization of 240.

Learning Objective #3: Reduce or simplify fractions.

✔ *Solved Problem #3*

3a. Reduce $\dfrac{10}{15}$ to its lowest terms.

$$\frac{10}{15} = \frac{2 \cdot \cancel{5}}{3 \cdot \cancel{5}} = \frac{2}{3}$$

3b. Reduce $\dfrac{13}{15}$ to its lowest terms.

13 and 15 share no common factors (other than 1).

Therefore, $\dfrac{13}{15}$ is already reduced to its lowest terms.

✎ *Pencil Problem #3* ✎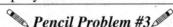

3a. Reduce $\dfrac{35}{50}$ to its lowest terms.

3b. Reduce $\dfrac{120}{86}$ to its lowest terms.

Learning Objective #4: Multiply fractions.

✔ *Solved Problem #4*

4a. Multiply $\dfrac{4}{11} \cdot \dfrac{2}{3}$.

If possible, reduce the product to its lowest terms.

$$\frac{4}{11} \cdot \frac{2}{3} = \frac{4 \cdot 2}{11 \cdot 3}$$
$$= \frac{8}{33}$$

✎ *Pencil Problem #4* ✎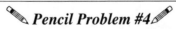

4a. Multiply $\dfrac{3}{8} \cdot \dfrac{7}{11}$.

If possible, reduce the product to its lowest terms.

Copyright © 2017 Pearson Education, Inc.

4b. Multiply $\left(3\dfrac{2}{5}\right)\left(1\dfrac{1}{2}\right)$.

If possible, reduce the product to its lowest terms.

$$\left(3\dfrac{2}{5}\right)\left(1\dfrac{1}{2}\right) = \dfrac{17}{5} \cdot \dfrac{3}{2}$$

$$= \dfrac{51}{10}$$

$$= 5\dfrac{1}{10}$$

4b. Multiply $\left(3\dfrac{3}{4}\right)\left(1\dfrac{3}{5}\right)$.

If possible, reduce the product to its lowest terms.

Learning Objective #5: Divide fractions.

✔ Solved Problem #5

✎ Pencil Problem #5✎

5a. Divide $\dfrac{5}{4} \div \dfrac{3}{8}$.

$$\dfrac{5}{4} \div \dfrac{3}{8} = \dfrac{5}{4} \cdot \dfrac{8}{3}$$

$$= \dfrac{5}{\cancel{4}} \cdot \dfrac{\cancel{4} \cdot 2}{3}$$

$$= \dfrac{10}{3}$$

$$= 3\dfrac{1}{3}$$

5a. Divide $\dfrac{7}{6} \div \dfrac{5}{3}$.

5b. Divide $3\dfrac{3}{8} \div 2\dfrac{1}{4}$.

$$3\dfrac{3}{8} \div 2\dfrac{1}{4} = \dfrac{27}{8} \div \dfrac{9}{4}$$

$$= \dfrac{27}{8} \cdot \dfrac{4}{9}$$

$$= \dfrac{\cancel{9} \cdot 3 \cdot \cancel{4}}{\cancel{4} \cdot 2 \cdot \cancel{9}}$$

$$= \dfrac{3}{2}$$

$$= 1\dfrac{1}{2}$$

5b. Divide $6\dfrac{3}{5} \div 1\dfrac{1}{10}$.

Learning Objective #6: Add and subtract fractions with identical denominators.

✔ Solved Problem #6

6a. Perform the indicated operation: $\dfrac{2}{11}+\dfrac{3}{11}$

$$\dfrac{2}{11}+\dfrac{3}{11}=\dfrac{2+3}{11}$$
$$=\dfrac{5}{11}$$

✎ Pencil Problem #6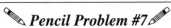

6a. Perform the indicated operation: $\dfrac{7}{12}+\dfrac{1}{12}$

6b. Perform the indicated operation: $\dfrac{5}{6}-\dfrac{1}{6}$

$$\dfrac{5}{6}-\dfrac{1}{6}=\dfrac{4}{6}$$
$$=\dfrac{2}{3}$$

6b. Perform the indicated operation: $\dfrac{11}{18}-\dfrac{4}{18}$

Learning Objective #7: Add and subtract fractions with unlike denominators.

✔ Solved Problem #7

7a. Perform the indicated operation: $\dfrac{1}{2}+\dfrac{3}{5}$

$$\dfrac{1}{2}+\dfrac{3}{5}=\dfrac{1\cdot5}{2\cdot5}+\dfrac{3\cdot2}{5\cdot2}$$
$$=\dfrac{5}{10}+\dfrac{6}{10}$$
$$=\dfrac{5+6}{10}$$
$$=\dfrac{11}{10}$$
$$=1\dfrac{1}{10}$$

✎ Pencil Problem #7

7a. Perform the indicated operation: $\dfrac{3}{8}+\dfrac{5}{12}$

Copyright © 2017 Pearson Education, Inc.

7b. Perform the indicated operation: $3\dfrac{1}{6} - 1\dfrac{11}{12}$

7b. Perform the indicated operation: $3\dfrac{3}{4} - 2\dfrac{1}{3}$

$$
\begin{aligned}
3\frac{1}{6} - 1\frac{11}{12} &= \frac{19}{6} - \frac{23}{12} \\
&= \frac{19 \cdot 2}{6 \cdot 2} - \frac{23}{12} \\
&= \frac{38}{12} - \frac{23}{12} \\
&= \frac{15}{12} \\
&= \frac{5}{4} \\
&= 1\frac{1}{4}
\end{aligned}
$$

Learning Objective #8: Solve problems involving fractions in algebra.

✔ *Solved Problem #8*

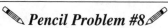 *Pencil Problem #8*

8a. Determine whether the given number is a solution of the equation.

$$x - \frac{2}{9}x = 1; \quad 1\frac{2}{7}$$

8a. Determine whether the given number is a solution of the equation.

$$\frac{2}{9}y + \frac{1}{3}y = \frac{3}{7}; \quad \frac{27}{35}$$

$$
\begin{aligned}
x - \frac{2}{9}x &= 1 \\
1\frac{2}{7} - \frac{2}{9}\left(1\frac{2}{7}\right) &= 1 \\
\frac{9}{7} - \frac{2}{9}\left(\frac{9}{7}\right) &= 1 \\
\frac{9}{7} - \frac{2}{7} &= 1 \\
\frac{7}{7} &= 1 \\
1 &= 1, \ \text{true}
\end{aligned}
$$

The given fraction is a solution.

8b. Translate from English to an algebraic expression or equation, whichever is appropriate. Let the variable x represent the number.

$$\frac{2}{3} \text{ of a number decreased by 6.}$$

$$\frac{2}{3}(x-6)$$

8b. Translate from English to an algebraic expression or equation, whichever is appropriate. Let the variable x represent the number.

$$\text{A number decreased by } \frac{1}{4} \text{ of itself.}$$

8c. The temperature on a warm spring day is 77°F. Use the formula $C = \frac{5}{9}(F-32)$ to find the equivalent temperature on the Celsius scale.

$$C = \frac{5}{9}(F-32)$$

$$C = \frac{5}{9}(77-32)$$

$$= \frac{5}{9}(45)$$

$$= 25$$

77°F is equivalent to 25°C.

8c. The temperature on a cool fall day is 68°F. Use the formula $C = \frac{5}{9}(F-32)$ to find the equivalent temperature on the Celsius scale.

Answers for Pencil Problems *(Textbook Exercise references in parentheses)*:

1a. $\frac{38}{5}$ *(1.2 #3)*   **1b.** $8\frac{4}{9}$ *(1.2 #9)*   **2.** $2 \cdot 2 \cdot 2 \cdot 2 \cdot 3 \cdot 5$ *(1.2 #27)*   **3a.** $\frac{7}{10}$ *(1.2 #33)*   **3b.** $\frac{60}{43}$ *(1.2 #39)*

4a. $\frac{21}{88}$ *(1.2 #43)*   **4b.** 6 *(1.2 #51)*   **5a.** $\frac{7}{10}$ *(1.2 #61)*   **5b.** 6 *(1.2 #65)*

6a. $\frac{2}{3}$ *(1.2 #69)*   **6b.** $\frac{7}{18}$ *(1.2 #83)*   **7a.** $\frac{19}{24}$ *(1.2 #81)*   **7b.** $\frac{17}{12}$ or $1\frac{5}{12}$ *(1.2 #89)*

8a. solution *(1.2 #97)*   **8b.** $x - \frac{1}{4}x$ *(1.2 #105)*   **8c.** 20°C *(1.2 #123)*

Homework:

☐ **Review the Section** 1.2 **summary** that begins on page 103 of the textbook.

☐ **Insert your homework** into this section of the *Learning Guide*. Show all work neatly and check your answers. Strive to work through difficulties when possible, making note of any exercises where you need additional help. Remember, even if your instructor assigns homework through *MyMathLab*, you should still write out your work.

Copyright © 2017 Pearson Education, Inc.

Section 1.3
The Real Numbers

The Golden Rectangle
Which of the following rectangles do you feel is most visually pleasing?

| #1 | #2 | #3 |

Did you know that the ancient Greeks believed that the most visually pleasing rectangles needed to have the ratio of the width to the height be exactly $\sqrt{5}+1$ to 2?

In this section of your textbook, you will explore numbers such as $\sqrt{5}$.
And by the way, rectangle #2 above has the dimensions of the golden rectangle.

First Steps:

☐ **Take comprehensive notes** from your instructor's lecture and insert your notes into this section of the *Learning Guide*. Be sure to write down all examples, definitions, and other key concepts. Additional learning resources include the *Video Lecture Series*, the *PowerPoints*, and Section 1.3 of your textbook which begins on page 32.

☐ Complete the **Concept and Vocabulary Check** on page 41 of the textbook.

Guided Practice:

☐ Review each of the following **Solved Problems** and complete each **Pencil Problem**.

Learning Objective #1: Define the sets that make up the real numbers.	
✔ **Solved Problem #1**	✎ **Pencil Problem #1**
1a. Write a positive or negative integer that describes the following situation. A debt of $500 −500	**1a.** Write a positive or negative integer that describes the following situation. A gain of 8 pounds
1b. Write a positive or negative integer that describes the following situation. 282 feet below sea level. −282	**1b.** Write a positive or negative integer that describes the following situation. A bank withdrawal of $3000

Learning Objective #2: Graph numbers on a number line.

✔ *Solved Problem #2*

2a. Graph: -4

(a)

$$\begin{array}{c} \bullet \\ \hline -5\ -4\ -3\ -2\ -1\ \ 0\ \ 1\ \ 2\ \ 3\ \ 4\ \ 5 \end{array}$$

2b. Graph: -1.2

(b)

$$\begin{array}{c} \bullet \\ \hline -5\ -4\ -3\ -2\ -1\ \ 0\ \ 1\ \ 2\ \ 3\ \ 4\ \ 5 \end{array}$$

✎ *Pencil Problem #2* ✎

2a. Graph: 2

2b. Graph: $-\dfrac{16}{5}$

Learning Objective #3: Express rational numbers as decimals.

✔ *Solved Problem #3*

3a. Express the rational number as a decimal: $\dfrac{3}{8}$

$$\begin{array}{r} 0.375 \\ 8\overline{)3.000} \\ \underline{24} \\ 60 \\ \underline{56} \\ 40 \\ \underline{40} \\ 0 \end{array}$$

$\dfrac{3}{8} = 0.375$

3b. Express the rational number as a decimal: $\dfrac{5}{11}$

$$\begin{array}{r} 0.454... \\ 11\overline{)5.000...} \\ \underline{44} \\ 60 \\ \underline{55} \\ 50 \\ \underline{44} \\ 60 \end{array}$$

$\dfrac{5}{11} = 0.\overline{45}$

✎ *Pencil Problem #3* ✎

3a. Express the rational number as a decimal: $\dfrac{7}{8}$

3b. Express the rational number as a decimal: $\dfrac{9}{11}$

Copyright © 2017 Pearson Education, Inc.

Learning Objective #4: Classify numbers as belonging to one or more sets of the real numbers.

✔ *Solved Problem #4*	✎ *Pencil Problem #4*✎

4. List all numbers from the given set that are:
a. natural numbers, **b.** whole numbers, **c.** integers,
d. rational numbers, **e.** irrational numbers,
f. real numbers.

$$\left\{ -9, -1.3, 0, 0.\overline{3}, \frac{\pi}{2}, \sqrt{9}, \sqrt{10} \right\}$$

a. $\sqrt{9}$

b. $0, \sqrt{9}$

c. $-9, 0, \sqrt{9}$

d. $-9, -1.3, 0, 0.\overline{3}, \sqrt{9}$

e. $\frac{\pi}{2}, \sqrt{10}$

f. $-9, -1.3, 0, 0.\overline{3}, \frac{\pi}{2}, \sqrt{9}, \sqrt{10}$

4. List all numbers from the given set that are:
a. natural numbers, **b.** whole numbers, **c.** integers,
d. rational numbers, **e.** irrational numbers,
f. real numbers.

$$\left\{ -11, -\frac{5}{6}, 0, 0.75, \sqrt{5}, \pi, \sqrt{64} \right\}$$

Learning Objective #5: Understand and use inequality symbols.

✔ *Solved Problem #5*	✎ *Pencil Problem #5*✎

5a. Insert either $<$ or $>$ to make the statement true.
$$-19 \quad -6$$

Since -19 is to the left of -6 on the number line,
then $-19 < -6$.

5a. Insert either $<$ or $>$ to make the statement true.
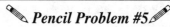
$$-\pi \quad -3.5$$

5b. Determine if the inequality is true or false.
$$-2 \geq -2$$

Because $-2 = -2$ is true,
then $-2 \geq -2$ is true.

5b. Determine if the inequality is true or false.
$$0 \geq -6$$

5c. Determine if the inequality is true or false.
$$-4 \geq 1$$

Because neither $-4 > 1$ nor $-4 = 1$ is true,
then $-4 \geq 1$ is false.

5c. Determine if the inequality is true or false.
$$-17 \geq 6$$

Learning Objective #6: Find the absolute value of a real number.	
✔ **Solved Problem #6**	✎ **Pencil Problem #6**
6a. Find the absolute value: $\left\|-4\right\|$	**6a.** Find the absolute value: $\left\|-7\right\|$
-4 is 4 units from 0. Thus $\left\|-4\right\| = 4$.	
6b. Find the absolute value: $\left\|-\sqrt{2}\right\|$	**6b.** Find the absolute value: $\left\|\dfrac{5}{6}\right\|$
$-\sqrt{2}$ is $\sqrt{2}$ units from 0. Thus $\left\|-\sqrt{2}\right\| = \sqrt{2}$.	

Answers for Pencil Problems *(Textbook Exercise references in parentheses)*:

1a. 8 *(1.3 #3)*   **1b.** -3000 *(1.3 #5)*

2a. 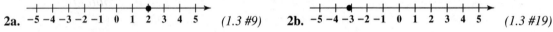 *(1.3 #9)*   **2b.** *(1.3 #19)*

3a. 0.875 *(1.3 #25)*   **3b.** $0.\overline{81}$ *(1.3 #27)*

4a. $\sqrt{64}$ *(1.3 #35)*   **4b.** $0, \sqrt{64}$ *(1.3 #35)*   **4c.** $-11, 0, \sqrt{64}$ *(1.3 #35)*

4d. $-11, -\dfrac{5}{6}, 0, 0.75, \sqrt{64}$ *(1.3 #35)*   **4e.** $\sqrt{5}, \pi$ *(1.3 #35)*   **4f.** $-11, -\dfrac{5}{6}, 0, 0.75, \sqrt{5}, \pi, \sqrt{64}$ *(1.3 #35)*

5a. $-\pi > -3.5$ *(1.3 #61)*   **5b.** true *(1.3 #67)*   **5c.** false *(1.3 #69)*

6a. 7 *(1.3 #73)*   **6b.** $\dfrac{5}{6}$ *(1.3 #75)*

Homework:

☐ **Review the Section 1.3 summary** on page 104 of the textbook.

☐ **Insert your homework** into this section of the *Learning Guide*. Show all work neatly and check your answers. Strive to work through difficulties when possible, making note of any exercises where you need additional help. Remember, even if your instructor assigns homework through *MyMathLab*, you should still write out your work.

Copyright © 2017 Pearson Education, Inc.

Widening the World Wide Web

In the time it took for the number of internet users in the United States to double, the number of internet users worldwide more than quadrupled.

In the Exercise Set of this section of your textbook, you will simplify, and then utilize, formulas that model these changes in the number of Internet users.

First Steps:

☐ **Take comprehensive notes** from your instructor's lecture and insert your notes into this section of the *Learning Guide*. Be sure to write down all examples, definitions, and other key concepts. Additional learning resources include the *Video Lecture Series*, the *PowerPoints*, and Section 1.4 of your textbook which begins on page 44.

☐ Complete the ***Concept and Vocabulary Check*** on page 53 of the textbook.

Guided Practice:

☐ Review each of the following ***Solved Problems*** and complete each ***Pencil Problem***.

Learning Objective #1: Understand and use the vocabulary of algebraic expressions.	
✔ *Solved Problem #1*	✎ *Pencil Problem #1* ✎

1. Use the algebraic expression

$$6x + 2x + 11$$

to answer the following questions.

1. Use the algebraic expression

$$x + 2 + 5x$$

to answer the following questions.

1a. How many terms are in the algebraic expression?

There are 3 terms.

1a. How many terms are in the algebraic expression?

1b. What is the coefficient of the first term?

6 is the coefficient of the first term.

1b. What is the coefficient of the first term?

1c. What is the constant term?

11 is the constant term.

1c. What is the constant term?

1d. What are the like terms in the algebraic expression?

$6x$ and $2x$ are like terms.

1d. What are the like terms in the algebraic expression?

Copyright © 2017 Pearson Education, Inc.

Learning Objective #2: Use commutative properties.

✔ **Solved Problem #2**

2a. Use the commutative property of addition to write an equivalent algebraic expression of $x+14$.

$14+x$

2b. Use the commutative property of multiplication to write an equivalent algebraic expression of $7y$.

$y7$

✎ **Pencil Problem #2**✎

2a. Use the commutative property of addition to write an equivalent algebraic expression of $y+4$.

2b. Use the commutative property of multiplication to write an equivalent algebraic expression of $9x$.

Learning Objective #3: Use associative properties.

✔ **Solved Problem #3**

3a. Simplify: $8+(x+4)$

$$8+(x+4)=8+(4+x)$$
$$=(8+4)+x$$
$$=12+x \text{ or } x+12$$

3b. Simplify: $6(5x)$

$$6(5x)=(6\cdot5)x$$
$$=30x$$

✎ **Pencil Problem #3**✎

3a. Simplify: $7+(5+x)$

3b. Simplify: $7(4x)$

Learning Objective #4: Use the distributive property.

✔ **Solved Problem #4**

4a. Multiply: $5(x+3)$

$$5(x+3)=5\cdot x+5\cdot3$$
$$=5x+15$$

✎ **Pencil Problem #4**✎

4a. Multiply: $3(x-2)$

Copyright © 2017 Pearson Education, Inc.

4b. Multiply: $6(4y+7)$

$$6(4y+7) = 6 \cdot 4y + 6 \cdot 7$$
$$= 24y + 42$$

4b. Multiply: $2(4x-5)$

Learning Objective #5: Combine like terms.

✔ *Solved Problem #5*

✎ *Pencil Problem #5* ✎

5a. Combine like terms: $7x+3x$

$$7x+3x = (7+3)x$$
$$= 10x$$

5a. Combine like terms: $7x+10x$

5b. Combine like terms: $9a-4a$

$$9a-4a = (9-4)a$$
$$= 5a$$

5b. Combine like terms: $11a-3a$

5c. Simplify: $9x+6y+5x+2y$

$$9x+6y+5x+2y = 9x+5x+6y+2y$$
$$= (9+5)x + (6+2)y$$
$$= 14x + 8y$$

5c. Simplify: $11a+12+3a+2$

Copyright © 2017 Pearson Education, Inc.

Learning Objective #6: Simplify algebraic expressions.

✔ **Solved Problem #6**	✎ *Pencil Problem #6* ✐
6a. Simplify: $7(2x+3)+11x$	**6a.** Simplify: $5(3x+2)-4$

$$7(2x+3)+11x = 7 \cdot 2x + 7 \cdot 3 + 11x$$
$$= 14x + 21 + 11x$$
$$= (14x + 11x) + 21$$
$$= 25x + 21$$

6b. Simplify: $7(4x+3y)+2(5x+y)$	**6b.** Simplify: $7(3a+2b)+5(4a+2b)$

$$7(4x+3y)+2(5x+y) = 7 \cdot 4x + 7 \cdot 3y + 2 \cdot 5x + 2 \cdot y$$
$$= 28x + 21y + 10x + 2y$$
$$= (28x + 10x) + (21y + 2y)$$
$$= 38x + 23y$$

Answers for Pencil Problems *(Textbook Exercise references in parentheses)*:

1a. 3 *(1.4 #3a)*　**1b.** 1 *(1.4 #3b)*　**1c.** 2 *(1.4 #3c)*　**1d.** x and $5x$ *(1.4 #3d)*

2a. $4+y$ *(1.4 #7)*　**2b.** $x9$ *(1.4 #15)*　**3a.** $12+x$ *(1.4 #23)*　**3b.** $28x$ *(1.4 #25)*

4a. $3x-6$ *(1.4 #35)*　**4b.** $8x-10$ *(1.4 #37)*　**5a.** $17x$ *(1.4 #47)*　**5b.** $8a$ *(1.4 #49)*

5c. $14a+14$ *(1.4 #57)*　**6a.** $15x+6$ *(1.4 #59)*　**6b.** $41a+24b$ *(1.4 #63)*

Homework:

☐ **Review the Section 1.4 summary** on page 105 of the textbook.

☐ **Insert your homework** into this section of the *Learning Guide*. Show all work neatly and check your answers. Strive to work through difficulties when possible, making note of any exercises where you need additional help. Remember, even if your instructor assigns homework through *MyMathLab*, you should still write out your work.

　Copyright © 2017 Pearson Education, Inc.

Section 1.5
Addition of Real Numbers

First and Ten!!!

The rules of football can be confusing sometimes.
One of the objectives that is usually obvious to most people is that your team's offense desires to move the ball down field.

One of the application exercises in this section of your textbook uses the concept of adding signed numbers to analyze the result of several consecutive plays.

First Steps:

☐ **Take comprehensive notes** from your instructor's lecture and insert your notes into this section of the *Learning Guide*. Be sure to write down all examples, definitions, and other key concepts. Additional learning resources include the *Video Lecture Series*, the *PowerPoints*, and Section 1.5 of your textbook which begins on page 56.

☐ Complete the ***Concept and Vocabulary Check*** on page 62 of the textbook.

Guided Practice:

☐ Review each of the following ***Solved Problems*** and complete each ***Pencil Problem***.

Learning Objective #1: Add numbers with a number line.	
✔ *Solved Problem #1*	✎ *Pencil Problem #1*✎

1a. Find the sum using a number line: $4+(-7)$

Start at 4 and move 7 units to the left.

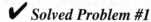

Thus, $4+(-7)=-3$

1a. Find the sum using a number line: $7+(-3)$

1b. Find the sum using a number line: $-1+(-3)$

Start at -1 and move 3 units to the left.

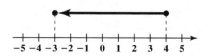

Thus, $-1+(-3)=-4$

1b. Find the sum using a number line: $-2+(-5)$

Copyright © 2017 Pearson Education, Inc.

1c. Find the sum using a number line: $-5+3$

Start at -5 and move 3 units to the right.

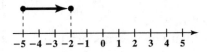

$$-5 \quad -4 \quad -3 \quad -2 \quad -1 \quad 0 \quad 1 \quad 2 \quad 3 \quad 4 \quad 5$$

Thus, $-5+3 = -2$

1c. Find the sum using a number line: $3+(-3)$

Learning Objective #2: Find sums using identity and inverse properties.

✔ Solved Problem #2

2. Use the Inverse Property of Addition to add:
$6+(-6)$

The sum of a real number and its additive inverse, or opposite, gives 0, the additive identity.

$6+(-6) = 0$

✎ Pencil Problem #2 ✎

2. Use the Identity Property of Addition to add:
$-7+0$

Learning Objective #3: Add numbers without a number line.

✔ Solved Problem #3

3a. Add without using a number line: $-10+(-25)$

$-10+(-25) = -35$

✎ Pencil Problem #3 ✎

3a. Add without using a number line: $-8+(-10)$

3b. Add without using a number line: $-\dfrac{2}{3}+\left(-\dfrac{1}{6}\right)$

$$-\frac{2}{3}+\left(-\frac{1}{6}\right) = -\frac{4}{6}+\left(-\frac{1}{6}\right)$$
$$= -\frac{5}{6}$$

3b. Add without using a number line: $\dfrac{9}{10}+\left(-\dfrac{3}{5}\right)$

Copyright © 2017 Pearson Education, Inc.

3c. Add without using a number line: $-0.4 + 1.6$

$-0.4 + 1.6 = 1.2$

3c. Add without using a number line: $-3.6 + (-2.1)$

Learning Objective #4: Use addition rules to simplify algebraic expressions.

✔ *Solved Problem #4*

4a. Simplify: $-20x + 3x$

$$-20x + 3x = (-20 + 3)x$$
$$= -17x$$

✎ *Pencil Problem #4*✎

4a. Simplify: $25y + (-12y)$

4b. Simplify: $3y + (-10z) + (-10y) + 16z$

$3y + (-10z) + (-10y) + 16z$
$= 3y + (-10y) + (-10z) + 16z$
$= [3 + (-10)]y + [(-10) + 16]z$
$= -7y + 6z$

4b. Simplify: $4y + (-13z) + (-10y) + 17z$

4c. Simplify: $5(2x + 3) + (-30x)$

$5(2x + 3) + (-30x) = 10x + 15 + (-30x)$
$= 10x + (-30x) + 15$
$= [10 + (-30)]x + 15$
$= -20x + 15$

4c. Simplify: $8(4y + 3) + (-35y)$

Learning Objective #5: Solve applied problems using a series of additions.

✔ Solved Problem #5

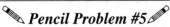 Pencil Problem #5

5. The water level of a reservoir is measured over a five-month period. During this time, the level rose 2 feet, then fell 4 feet, then rose 1 foot, then fell 5 feet, and then rose 3 feet. What was the change in the water level at the end of the five months?

5. The temperature at 8:00 a.m. was $-7°F$.

By noon it had risen $15°F$, but by 4:00 p.m. it had fallen $5°F$.

What was the temperature at 4:00 p.m.?

the level rose 2 feet: 2
then fell 4 feet: -4
then rose 1 foot: 1
then fell 5 feet: -5
and then rose 3 feet: 3

$$2+(-4)+1+(-5)+3 = (2+1+3)+\big[(-4)+(-5)\big]$$
$$= 6+(-9)$$
$$= -3$$

At the end of 5 months the water level was down 3 feet.

Answers for Pencil Problems *(Textbook Exercise references in parentheses)*:

1a. 4 *(1.5 #1)*   **1b.** -7 *(1.5 #3)*   **1c.** 0 *(1.5 #7)*

2. -7 *(1.5 #9)*

3a. -18 *(1.5 #15)*   **3b.** $\dfrac{3}{10}$ *(1.5 #31)*   **3c.** -5.7 *(1.5 #29)*

4a. $13y$ *(1.5 #49)*   **4b.** $-6y+4z$ *(1.5 #53)*   **4c.** $-3y+24$ *(1.5 #59)*

5. $3°F$ *(1.5 #75)*

Homework:

☐ **Review the Section 1.5 summary** that begins on page 105 of the textbook.

☐ **Insert your homework** into this section of the *Learning Guide*. Show all work neatly and check your answers. Strive to work through difficulties when possible, making note of any exercises where you need additional help. Remember, even if your instructor assigns homework through *MyMathLab*, you should still write out your work.

     Copyright © 2017 Pearson Education, Inc.

Section 1.6
Subtraction of Real Numbers

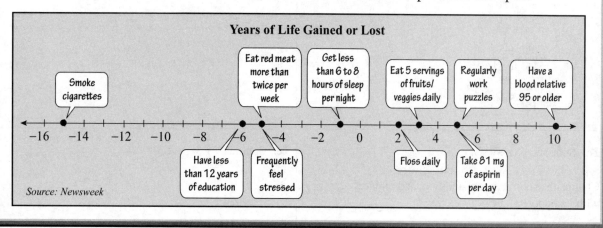

Stretching and Shrinking One's Life Span

Life expectancy for the average American man is 75.2 years.
Life expectancy for the average American woman is 80.4 years.

The number line below, with points representing eight integers, indicates factors,
many within our control, that can stretch or shrink one's probable life span.

Years of Life Gained or Lost

Smoke cigarettes

Eat red meat more than twice per week

Get less than 6 to 8 hours of sleep per night

Eat 5 servings of fruits/veggies daily

Regularly work puzzles

Have a blood relative 95 or older

−16 −14 −12 −10 −8 −6 −4 −2 0 2 4 6 8 10

Have less than 12 years of education

Frequently feel stressed

Floss daily

Take 81 mg of aspirin per day

Source: Newsweek

First Steps:

☐ **Take comprehensive notes** from your instructor's lecture and insert your notes into this
section of the *Learning Guide*. Be sure to write down all examples, definitions, and other
key concepts. Additional learning resources include the *Video Lecture Series*, the
PowerPoints, and Section 1.6 of your textbook which begins on page 65.

☐ Complete the *Concept and Vocabulary Check* on page 70 of the textbook.

Guided Practice:

☐ Review each of the following *Solved Problems* and complete each *Pencil Problem*.

Learning Objective #1: Subtract real numbers.

✔ **Solved Problem #1**	✎ **Pencil Problem #1** ✎
1a. Subtract: $-7-(-2)$	**1a.** Subtract: $3-(-20)$

Change the subtraction to addition, and replace -2 with
its opposite, 2.

$$-7-(-2) = -7+2$$
$$= -5$$

1b. Subtract: $-\dfrac{3}{5}-\dfrac{1}{3}$

Change the subtraction to addition, and replace $\dfrac{1}{3}$ with

its opposite, $-\dfrac{1}{3}$.

$$-\dfrac{3}{5}-\dfrac{1}{3}=-\dfrac{3}{5}+\left(-\dfrac{1}{3}\right)$$
$$=-\dfrac{9}{15}+\left(-\dfrac{5}{15}\right)$$
$$=-\dfrac{14}{15}$$

1b. Subtract: $\dfrac{3}{7}-\dfrac{5}{7}$

1c. Subtract: $5\pi-(-2\pi)$

Change the subtraction to addition, and replace -2π with its opposite, 2π.

$$5\pi-(-2\pi)=5\pi+2\pi$$
$$=7\pi$$

1c. Subtract: $1.3-(-1.3)$

Learning Objective #2: Simplify a series of additions and subtractions.

✔ *Solved Problem #2*

2. Simplify: $10-(-12)-4-(-3)-6$

$$10-(-12)-4-(-3)-6$$
$$=10+12+(-4)+3+(-6)$$
$$=(10+12+3)+\left[(-4)+(-6)\right]$$
$$=25+(-10)$$
$$=15$$

✎ *Pencil Problem #2*✎

2. Simplify: $-23-11-(-7)+(-25)$

Copyright © 2017 Pearson Education, Inc.

Learning Objective #3: Use the definition of subtraction to identify terms.

✔ *Solved Problem #3*	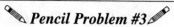 *Pencil Problem #3*
3. Identify the terms of the algebraic expression: $-6 + 4a - 7ab$	3. Identify the terms of the algebraic expression: $12x - 5xy - 4$
The terms are -6, $4a$, and $-7ab$.	

Learning Objective #4: Use the subtraction definition to simplify algebraic expressions.

✔ *Solved Problem #4*	✏ *Pencil Problem #4*
4a. Simplify: $4 + 2x - 9x$	**4a.** Simplify: $4 + 7y - 17y$

$$4 + 2x - 9x = 4 + (2 - 9)x$$
$$= 4 + [2 + (-9)]x$$
$$= 4 - 7x$$

4b. Simplify: $-3x - 10y - 6x + 14y$

4b. Simplify: $4 - 6b - 8 - 3b$

$$-3x - 10y - 6x + 14y = -3x - 6x - 10y + 14y$$
$$= (-3 - 6)x + (-10 + 14)y$$
$$= -9x + 4y$$

Learning Objective #5: Solve problems involving subtraction.

✔ *Solved Problem #5*	✎ *Pencil Problem #5*✎

5. This section of your Learning Guide opened by showing a number line that indicates various factors that can stretch or shrink one's probable lifespan. (The number line is copied below.)

Use that number line to determine the difference in the lifespan between a person who eats five servings of fruits/veggies daily and a person who frequently feels stressed.

$$3-(-5) = 3+5 = 8$$

The difference in lifespan is 8 years.

5. The peak of Mount Kilimanjaro, the highest point in Africa, is 19,321 feet above sea level. Qattara Depression, Egypt, one of the lowest points in Africa, is 436 feet below sea level.
What is the difference in elevation between the peak of Mount Kilimanjaro and the Qattara Depression?

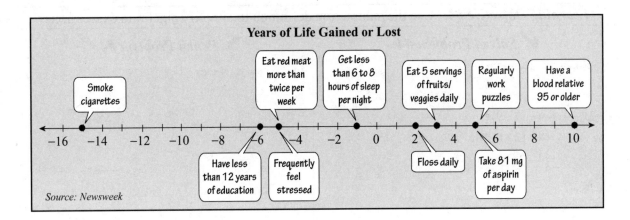

Answers for Pencil Problems *(Textbook Exercise references in parentheses)*:

1a. 23   *(1.6 #9)*   **1b.** $-\dfrac{2}{7}$ *(1.6 #27)*   **1c.** 2.6   *(1.6 #43)*

2. −52   *(1.6 #59)*

3. $12x$, $-5xy$, and −4   *(1.6 #71)*

4a. $4-10y$ *(1.6 #75)*   **4b.** $-4-9b$ *(1.6 #79)*

5. 19,757 feet   *(1.6 # 95)*

Homework:

☐ **Review the Section 1.6 summary** on page 106 of the textbook.

☐ **Insert your homework** into this section of the *Learning Guide*. Show all work neatly and check your answers. Strive to work through difficulties when possible, making note of any exercises where you need additional help. Remember, even if your instructor assigns homework through *MyMathLab*, you should still write out your work.

Copyright © 2017 Pearson Education, Inc.

Section 1.7
Multiplication and Division of Real Numbers

Do You Prefer a Large or Small Family?

The percentage of Americans that prefer small families (0, 1, or 2 children) is increasing. The percentage of Americans that prefer large families (3 or more children) is decreasing.

In the textbook's Exercise Set for this section, you will be presented with mathematical formulas that approximate how these preferences are changing over time.

First Steps:

☐ **Take comprehensive notes** from your instructor's lecture and insert your notes into this section of the *Learning Guide*. Be sure to write down all examples, definitions, and other key concepts. Additional learning resources include the *Video Lecture Series*, the *PowerPoints*, and Section 1.7 of your textbook which begins on page 74.

☐ Complete the *Concept and Vocabulary Check* on page 84 of the textbook.

Guided Practice:

☐ Review each of the following *Solved Problems* and complete each *Pencil Problem*.

Learning Objective #1: Multiply real numbers.	
✔ *Solved Problem #1*	✎ *Pencil Problem #1*
1a. Multiply: $-\dfrac{1}{3}\cdot\dfrac{4}{7}$ $-\dfrac{1}{3}\cdot\dfrac{4}{7}=-\dfrac{1\cdot4}{3\cdot7}$ $=-\dfrac{4}{21}$	**1a.** Multiply: $-\dfrac{3}{5}\cdot\left(-\dfrac{4}{7}\right)$
1b. Multiply: $(-12)(-3)$ $(-12)(-3)=36$	**1b.** Multiply: $5(-9)$
1c. Multiply: $(-543)(0)$ $(-543)(0)=0$	**1c.** Multiply: $0(-19)$

Copyright © 2017 Pearson Education, Inc.

Learning Objective #2: Multiply more than two real numbers.	
✔ *Solved Problem #2*	✏ *Pencil Problem #2* ✏
2a. Multiply: $(-2)(3)(-1)(4)$	**2a.** Multiply: $(-5)(-2)(3)$
$(-2)(3)(-1)(4) = 24$	
2b. Multiply: $(-1)(-3)(2)(-1)(5)$	**2b.** Multiply: $(-4)(-3)(-1)(6)$
$(-1)(-3)(2)(-1)(5) = -30$	

Learning Objective #3: Find multiplicative inverses.	
✔ *Solved Problem #3*	✏ *Pencil Problem #3* ✏
3a. Find the multiplicative inverse of 7.	**3a.** Find the multiplicative inverse of -10.
The multiplicative inverse of 7 is $\dfrac{1}{7}$ because $7 \cdot \dfrac{1}{7} = 1$. $\dfrac{1}{7}$	
3b. Find the multiplicative inverse of $-\dfrac{7}{13}$.	**3b.** Find the multiplicative inverse of $\dfrac{1}{5}$.
The multiplicative inverse of $-\dfrac{7}{13}$ is $-\dfrac{13}{7}$ because $\left(-\dfrac{7}{13}\right)\left(-\dfrac{13}{7}\right) = 1$. $-\dfrac{13}{7}$	

Learning Objective #4: Use the definition of division.	
✔ *Solved Problem #4*	✏ *Pencil Problem #4* ✏
4a. Use the definition of division to find the quotient: $-28 \div 7$	**4a.** Use the definition of division to find the quotient: $120 \div (-10)$
$\begin{aligned} -28 \div 7 &= -28 \cdot \dfrac{1}{7} \\ &= -4 \end{aligned}$	

Copyright © 2017 Pearson Education, Inc.

4b. Use the definition of division to find the quotient:

$$\frac{-16}{-2}$$

$$\frac{-16}{-2} = -16 \cdot \left(-\frac{1}{2}\right)$$
$$= 8$$

4b. Use the definition of division to find the quotient:

$$\frac{12}{-4}$$

Learning Objective #5: Divide real numbers.

✔ **Solved Problem #5**

5a. Divide: $-\dfrac{2}{3} \div \dfrac{5}{4}$

$$-\frac{2}{3} \div \frac{5}{4} = -\frac{2}{3} \cdot \frac{4}{5}$$
$$= -\frac{8}{15}$$

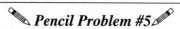 **Pencil Problem #5**

5a. Divide: $-\dfrac{1}{2} \div \left(-\dfrac{3}{5}\right)$

5b. Divide: $\dfrac{0}{-5}$

$$\frac{0}{-5} = 0$$

5b. Divide: $\dfrac{7}{0}$

Learning Objective #6: Simplify algebraic expressions involving multiplication.

✔ **Solved Problem #6**

6a. Simplify: $-7(3x-4)$

$$-7(3x-4) = -7(3x) - 7(-4)$$
$$= -21x + 28$$

Pencil Problem #6

6a. Simplify: $-4(2x-3)$

6b. Simplify: $4(3y-7) - (13y-2)$

$$4(3y-7) - (13y-2) = 12y - 28 - 13y + 2$$
$$= 12y - 13y - 28 + 2$$
$$= -1y - 26$$
$$= -y - 26$$

6b. Simplify: $4(2y-3) - (7y+2)$

Copyright © 2017 Pearson Education, Inc.

Learning Objective #7: Determine whether a number is a solution of an equation.	

✔ *Solved Problem #7*	✎ *Pencil Problem #7*
7. Determine whether –3 is a solution of $2x - 5 = 8x + 7$	7. Determine whether –4 is a solution of $-7y + 18 = -10y + 6$

$$2x - 5 = 8x + 7$$
$$2(-3) - 5 = 8(-3) + 7$$
$$-6 - 5 = -24 + 7$$
$$-11 = -17, \text{ false}$$

–3 is not a solution of the equation.

Learning Objective #8: Use mathematical models involving multiplication and division.	

✔ *Solved Problem #8*	✎ *Pencil Problem #8*
8. The data for doctorate degrees earned by men can be described by $M = -0.6n + 64.4$, where M is the percentage of doctorate degrees awarded to men n years after 1989. According to this mathematical model what percentage of doctorate degrees were received by men in 2014?	8. The percentage of American adults who smoked cigarettes is described by $C = -0.5x + 42$, where C is the percentage who smoked cigarettes n years after 1965. Use the mathematical model to project the percentage of American adults who will smoke cigarettes in 2019.

$$M = -0.6n + 64.4$$
$$M = -0.6(25) + 64.4$$
$$= -15 + 64.4$$
$$= 49.4$$

According to this model, 49.4% of doctorate degrees were awarded to men in 2014.

Answers for Pencil Problems *(Textbook Exercise references in parentheses)*:

1a. $\dfrac{12}{35}$ *(1.7 #15)*   **1b.** –45 *(1.7 #1)*   **1c.** 0 *(1.7 #9)*   **2a.** 30 *(1.7 #23)*   **2b.** –72 *(1.7 #25)*

3a. $-\dfrac{1}{10}$ *(1.7 #39)*   **3b.** 5 *(1.7 #37)*   **4a.** –12 *(1.7 #59)*   **4b.** –3 *(1.7 #47)*   **5a.** $\dfrac{5}{6}$ *(1.7 #69)*

5b. undefined *(1.7 #55)*   **6a.** $-8x + 12$ *(1.7 #89)*   **6b.** $y - 14$ *(1.7 #95)*   **7.** –4 is a solution *(1.7 #99)*

8. 15% *(1.7 #119b)*

Homework:

☐ **Review the Section 1.7 summary** that begins on page 106 of the textbook.

☐ **Insert your homework** into this section of the *Learning Guide*. Show all work neatly and check your answers. Strive to work through difficulties when possible, making note of any exercises where you need additional help. Remember, even if your instructor assigns homework through *MyMathLab*, you should still write out your work.

          Copyright © 2017 Pearson Education, Inc.

Section 1.8
Exponents and Order of Operations

High Cost of Cleaning Up Contaminants!

In Palo Alto, California, a government agency ordered computer-related companies to contribute to a pool of money to clean up underground water supplies. (The companies had stored toxic chemicals in leaking underground containers.)"

You will use the concepts discussed in this section of your textbook to calculate the costs for removing various percentages of the contaminants from the water supply.

First Steps:

☐ **Take comprehensive notes** from your instructor's lecture and insert your notes into this section of the *Learning Guide*. Be sure to write down all examples, definitions, and other key concepts. Additional learning resources include the *Video Lecture Series*, the *PowerPoints*, and Section 1.8 of your textbook which begins on page 88.

☐ Complete the *Concept and Vocabulary Check* on page 99 of the textbook.

Guided Practice:

☐ Review each of the following *Solved Problems* and complete each *Pencil Problem*.

Learning Objective #1: Evaluate exponential expressions.	
✔ *Solved Problem #1*	✎ *Pencil Problem #1* ✎
1a. Evaluate: 6^2 $6^2 = 6 \cdot 6$ $\quad = 36$	**1a.** Evaluate: 9^2
1b. Evaluate: $(-1)^4$ $(-1)^4 = (-1)(-1)(-1)(-1)$ $\quad = 1$	**1b.** Evaluate: $(-4)^3$
1c. Evaluate: -1^4 $-1^4 = -(1 \cdot 1 \cdot 1 \cdot 1)$ $\quad = -1$	**1c.** Evaluate: $(-5)^4$

Copyright © 2017 Pearson Education, Inc.

Learning Objective #2: Simplify algebraic expressions with exponents.	
✔ *Solved Problem #2*	✏ *Pencil Problem #2* ✏

2a. Simplify, if possible: $7x^3 + x^3$

$7x^3 + x^3 = 7x^3 + 1x^3$
$ = (7+1)x^3$
$ = 8x^3$

2a. Simplify, if possible: $26x^2 - 27x^2$

2b. Simplify, if possible: $10x^2 + 8x^3$

The terms $10x^2$ and $8x^3$ are not like terms because they have different variable factors, namely, x^2 and x^3.

$10x^2 + 8x^3$ cannot be simplified.

2b. Simplify, if possible: $5x^2 + 5x^3$

Learning Objective #3: Use the order of operations agreement.	
✔ *Solved Problem #3*	✏ *Pencil Problem #3* ✏

3a. Simplify: $20 + 4 \cdot 3 - 17$

$20 + 4 \cdot 3 - 17 = 20 + 12 - 17$
$ = 20 + 12 - 17$
$ = 15$

3a. Simplify: $7 + 6 \cdot 3$

3b. Simplify: $3 \cdot 2^2$

$3 \cdot 2^2 = 3 \cdot 4$
$ = 12$

3b. Simplify: $(4 \cdot 5)^2 - 4 \cdot 5^2$

3c. Simplify: $7^2 - 48 \div 4^2 \cdot 5 - 2$

$7^2 - 48 \div 4^2 \cdot 5 - 2 = 49 - 48 \div 16 \cdot 5 - 2$
$ = 49 - 3 \cdot 5 - 2$
$ = 49 - 15 - 2$
$ = 34 - 2$
$ = 32$

3c. Simplify: $8^2 - 16 \div 2^2 \cdot 4 - 3$

Copyright © 2017 Pearson Education, Inc.

3d. Simplify: $4[3(6-11)+5]$

$$4[3(6-11)+5] = 4[3(-5)+5]$$
$$= 4[-15+5]$$
$$= 4[-10]$$
$$= -40$$

3d. Simplify: $2[5+2(9-4)]$

3e. Simplify: $25 \div 5 + 3[4+2(7-9)^3]$

$$25 \div 5 + 3[4+2(7-9)^3] = 25 \div 5 + 3[4+2(-2)^3]$$
$$= 25 \div 5 + 3[4+2(-8)]$$
$$= 25 \div 5 + 3[4-16]$$
$$= 25 \div 5 + 3[-12]$$
$$= 5 + (-36)$$
$$= -31$$

3e. Simplify: $[7+3(2^3-1)] \div 21$

3f. Simplify: $\dfrac{5(4-9)+10\cdot 3}{2^3-1}$

$$\frac{5(4-9)+10\cdot 3}{2^3-1} = \frac{5(-5)+10\cdot 3}{8-1}$$
$$= \frac{-25+30}{7}$$
$$= \frac{5}{7}$$

3f. Simplify: $\dfrac{(-11)(-4)+2(-7)}{7-(-3)}$

3g. Evaluate $-x^2-4x$ for -5.

$$-x^2-4x = -(-5)^2-4(-5)$$
$$= -25+20$$
$$= -5$$

3g. Evaluate x^2+5x for $x=3$.

Copyright © 2017 Pearson Education, Inc.

Learning Objective #4: Evaluate mathematical models.

✔ Solved Problem #4

4. A company that manufactures running shoes has weekly fixed costs of \$300,000 and it costs \$30 to manufacture each pair of running shoes. The average cost per pair of running shoes, $\bar{C}$, for the company to manufacture x pairs per week is modeled by $\bar{C} = \dfrac{30x + 300,000}{x}$.

Find the average cost per pair of running shoes for the company to manufacture 10,000 pairs per week.

$$\bar{C} = \frac{30x + 300,000}{x}$$

$$\bar{C} = \frac{30(10,000) + 300,000}{10,000}$$

$$= \frac{300,000 + 300,000}{10,000}$$

$$= \frac{600,000}{10,000}$$

$$= 60$$

The average cost is \$60.

✎ Pencil Problem #4 ✎

4. A government agency ordered companies that had stored toxic chemicals in leaking underground containers to contribute to a pool of money to clean up underground water supplies.

The mathematical model $C = \dfrac{200x}{100 - x}$

describes the cost, C, in tens of thousands of dollars, for removing x percent of the contaminants.

Find the cost, in tens of thousands of dollars, for removing 80% of the contaminants.

Answers for Pencil Problems *(Textbook Exercise references in parentheses)*:

1a. 81 *(1.8 #1)*   **1b.** −64 *(1.8 #7)*   **1c.** 625 *(1.8 #9)*

2a. $-x^2$ *(1.8 #21)*   **2b.** $5x^2 + 5x^3$ cannot be simplified. *(1.8 #25)*

3a. 25 *(1.8 #29)*   **3b.** 300 *(1.8 #41)*   **3c.** 45 *(1.8 #37)*   **3d.** 30 *(1.8 #49)*

3e. $\dfrac{4}{3}$ *(1.8 #51)*   **3f.** 3 *(1.8 #57)*   **3g.** 24 *(1.8 #73)*   **4.** \$8,000,000 *(1.8 #101b)*

Homework:

☐ **Review the Section 1.8 summary** on page 107 of the textbook.

☐ **Insert your homework** into this section of the *Learning Guide*. Show all work neatly and check your answers. Strive to work through difficulties when possible, making note of any exercises where you need additional help. Remember, even if your instructor assigns homework through *MyMathLab*, you should still write out your work.

Copyright © 2017 Pearson Education, Inc.

Group Project for Chapter 1

One measure of physical fitness is your *resting heart rate*. Generally speaking, the more fit you are, the lower your resting heart rate. The best time to take this measurement is when you first awaken in the morning, before you get out of bed. Lie on your back with no body parts crossed and take your pulse in your neck or wrist. Use your index and second fingers and count your pulse beat for one full minute to get your resting heart rate. A resting heart rate under 48 to 57 indicates high fitness, 58 to 62, above average fitness, 63 to 70, average fitness, 71 to 82, below average fitness, and 83 or more, low fitness.

Another measure of physical fitness is your percentage of body fat. You can estimate your body fat using the following formulas:

For men: Body fat $= -98.42 + 4.15w - 0.082b$
For women: Body fat $= -76.76 + 4.15w - 0.082b$

where w = waist measurement, in inches, and b = total body weight, in pounds. Then divide your body fat by your total weight to get your body fat percentage. For men, less than 15% is considered athletic, 25% about average. For women, less than 22% is considered athletic, 30% about average.

Each group member should bring his or her age, resting heart rate, and body fat percentage to the group. Using the data, the group should create three graphs.

a. Create a graph that shows age and resting heart rate for group members.

b. Create a graph that shows age and body fat percentage for group members.

c. Create a graph that shows resting heart rate and body fat percentage for group members.

For each graph, select the style (line or bar) that is most appropriate.

Copyright © 2017 Pearson Education, Inc.

Getting Ready for the Chapter 1 Test

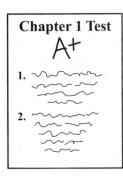

One of the best ways to prepare for a test is to stay on top of your studying, keeping up as your professor proceeds from section to section. Falling behind on one section often makes it difficult to understand the material in the following section. Never wait until the last minute to study for an exam.

Below are several actions that will help you stay organized as you prepare for your test.

How to prepare for your Chapter Test:

☐ **Write down any details that your instructor shares about the test.**
In addition to items such as location, date, time, and essentials to bring, be sure to listen carefully for specific information about the topics covered. Communicate with your instructor concerning any details that may be unclear to you.

☐ **Read the Chapter Summary that begins on page 102 of your textbook.**
Study the appropriate sections in the Chapter Summary. This summary contains the most important material in each section including, definitions, concepts, procedures, and examples.

☐ **Review your *Learning Guide*.**
Go back through the *Solved Problems* and *Pencil Problems* in this chapter of your *Learning Guide*. You may find it helpful to cover up solutions and work through the problems again.

☐ **Study your notes and homework.**
Read through your class notes that you took during this unit, and review the corresponding homework assignments.

☐ **Review quizzes and other feedback from your professor.**
Review any quizzes you have taken and be sure you understand any errors that you made. Seek help with any concepts that are still unclear.

☐ **Complete the Review Exercises that begin on page 108 of your textbook.**
Work the assigned problems from the Review Exercises. These exercises represent the most significant problems for each of the chapter's sections. The answers for all Review Exercises are in the back of your textbook.

☐ **Take the Chapter Test that begins on page 111 of your textbook.**
- Find a quiet place to take the Chapter Test.
- Do not use notes, index cards, or any resources other than those your instructor will allow during the actual test.
- After completing the entire test, check your answers in the back of the textbook.
- Watch the *Chapter Test Prep Video* to review any exercises you may have missed.

Copyright © 2017 Pearson Education, Inc.

Chapter 2.R Linear Equations and Inequalities in One Variable
Integrated Review

> **Learning Objectives**
> 1. Express rational numbers as decimals.
> 2. Graph numbers on a number line.
> 3. Understand and use inequality symbols.

Learning Objective #1: Express rational numbers as decimals.

✔ *Solved Problem #1*

1a. Express the rational number as a decimal: $\dfrac{3}{8}$

$$
\begin{array}{r}
0.375 \\
8\overline{)3.000} \\
\underline{24} \\
60 \\
\underline{56} \\
40 \\
\underline{40} \\
0
\end{array}
$$

$$\frac{3}{8} = 0.375$$

1b. Express the rational number as a decimal: $\dfrac{5}{11}$

$$
\begin{array}{r}
0.454... \\
11\overline{)5.000...} \\
\underline{44} \\
60 \\
\underline{55} \\
50 \\
\underline{44} \\
60
\end{array}
$$

$$\frac{5}{11} = 0.\overline{45}$$

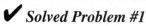 *Pencil Problem #1*

1a. Express the rational number as a decimal: $\dfrac{7}{8}$

1b. Express the rational number as a decimal: $\dfrac{9}{11}$

Learning Objective #2: Graph numbers on a number line.

✔ **Solved Problem #2**	✎ *Pencil Problem #2*✎

2a. Graph $\dfrac{3}{5}$ on a number line.

We use the fraction's denominator, 5, to divide the distance from 0 to 1 into 5 equal parts. Then we use the fraction's numerator, 2, to move 2 parts to the right.

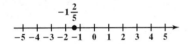

2a. Graph $\dfrac{-5}{7}$ on a number line.

2b. Graph $-1\dfrac{2}{5}$ on a number line.

The mixed number is between the consecutive integers –2 and –1. The denominator is 5, so we divide the distance between –2 and –1 into 5 equal parts. Then we use the fraction's numerator, 2, to move 2 parts to the left of –1. We move to the left because the given number is negative.

2b. Graph $-\dfrac{7}{4}$ on a number line.

Copyright © 2017 Pearson Education, Inc.

Learning Objective #3: Understand and use inequality symbols.

✔ *Solved Problem #3*	✎ *Pencil Problem #3* ✎
3a. Insert either < or > between the pair of decimals to make a true statement.	**3a.** Insert either <, >, or = between the pair of decimals to make a true statement.
5.769 5.771	0.089 0.1

5.7$\underline{6}$9 [?] 7.7$\underline{7}$1

Each corresponding digit is the same until the hundredths place (underlined).
Because $6 < 7$, then $5.769 < 7.771$.

3b. Insert either <, >, or = between the pair of decimals to make a true statement.	**3b.** Insert either <, >, or = between the pair of decimals to make a true statement.
−5.6 −5.06	−12.07 −12.7

-5.6 [?] -5.06

Notice that -5.6 has one decimal place, whereas -5.06 has two. Therefore, we write a 0 digit at the end of -5.6 to get -5.60.

$-5.\underline{6}0$ [?] $-5.\underline{0}6$

Each corresponding digit is the same until the tenths place (underlined). Because $6 > 0$, we conclude $-5.6 < -5.06$. Notice that the smaller digit determines the greater negative number.

Answers for Pencil Problems:

1a. 0.875 **1b.** $0.\overline{81}$ **2a.**

$-\frac{5}{7}$

$\begin{array}{c}\text{—|—|—|—|—|—●|—|—|—|—|—|—→}\\ -5\ -4\ -3\ -2\ -1\quad 0\quad 1\quad 2\quad 3\quad 4\quad 5\end{array}$

2b.

$-\frac{7}{4}$

$\begin{array}{c}\text{—|—|—|—●|—|—|—|—|—|—|—|—→}\\ -5\ -4\ -3\ -2\ -1\quad 0\quad 1\quad 2\quad 3\quad 4\quad 5\end{array}$

3a. <   **3b.** >

Copyright © 2017 Pearson Education, Inc.

Section 2.1
The Addition Property of Equality

Up, Up, and Away!

U.S. high schools are experiencing grade inflation.

In 1980 about 27% of college freshman had an average grade of A in high school.
By 2013 that percentage had risen to 53%.

In the Exercise Set of this section of your textbook, you will find a mathematical
formula that can be used to predict where grades are headed in the future.

First Steps:

☐ **Take comprehensive notes** from your instructor's lecture and insert your notes into this
section of the *Learning Guide*. Be sure to write down all examples, definitions, and other
key concepts. Additional learning resources include the *Video Lecture Series*, the
PowerPoints, and Section 2.1 of your textbook which begins on page 114.

☐ Complete the ***Concept and Vocabulary Check*** on page 120 of the textbook.

Guided Practice:

☐ Review each of the following ***Solved Problems*** and complete each ***Pencil Problem***.

Learning Objective #1: Identify linear equations in one variable.	
✔ ***Solved Problem #1***	***Pencil Problem #1***
Identify the linear equations in one variable.	Identify the linear equations in one variable.
1a. $3x + 7 = 9$	**1a.** $x - 9 = 13$
Linear; because the equation is of the form $ax + b = c$, with $a = 3$, $b = 7$, and $c = 9$.	
1b. $|x + 2| = 5$	**1b.** $x^2 - 9 = 13$
Nonlinear; because of the absolute value bars around x.	
1c. $x = 6.8$	**1c.** $\dfrac{9}{x} = 13$
Linear; because the equation, which can be written as $1x + 0 = 6.8$, is of the form $ax + b = c$, with $a = 1$, $b = 0$, and $c = 6.8$.	

Learning Objective #2: Use the addition property of equality to solve equations.	
✔ *Solved Problem #2*	✎ *Pencil Problem #2* ✎

2a. Solve and check: $x - 5 = 12$

$x - 5 = 12$

$x - 5 + 5 = 12 + 5$

$x + 0 = 17$

$x = 17$

The solution set is $\{17\}$.

Check: $x - 5 = 12$

$17 - 5 = 12$

$12 = 12$, true

2b. Solve and check: $z + 2.8 = 5.09$

$z + 2.8 = 5.09$

$z + 2.8 - 2.8 = 5.09 - 2.8$

$z + 0 = 2.29$

$z = 2.29$

The solution set is $\{2.29\}$.

Check: $z + 2.8 = 5.09$

$2.29 + 2.8 = 5.09$

$5.09 = 5.09$, true

2c. Solve: $-\dfrac{1}{2} = x - \dfrac{3}{4}$

$-\dfrac{1}{2} = x - \dfrac{3}{4}$

$-\dfrac{1}{2} + \dfrac{3}{4} = x - \dfrac{3}{4} + \dfrac{3}{4}$

$-\dfrac{2}{4} + \dfrac{3}{4} = x$

$\dfrac{1}{4} = x$

The solution set is $\left\{\dfrac{1}{4}\right\}$.

2a. Solve and check: $x - 4 = 19$

2b. Solve and check: $7 + z = 11$

2c. Solve: $t + \dfrac{5}{6} = -\dfrac{7}{12}$

Copyright © 2017 Pearson Education, Inc.

2d. Solve and check: $8y + 7 - 7y - 10 = 6 + 4$

$$8y + 7 - 7y - 10 = 6 + 4$$
$$y - 3 = 10$$
$$y - 3 + 3 = 10 + 3$$
$$y = 13$$

The solution set is $\{13\}$.

Check:
$$8y + 7 - 7y - 10 = 6 + 4$$
$$8(13) + 7 - 7(13) - 10 = 6 + 4$$
$$104 + 7 - 91 - 10 = 10$$
$$111 - 101 = 10$$
$$10 = 10, \text{ true}$$

2d. Solve and check: $6y + 3 - 5y = 14$

2e. Solve and check: $7x = 12 + 6x$

$$7x = 12 + 6x$$
$$7x - 6x = 12 + 6x - 6x$$
$$x = 12$$

The solution set is $\{12\}$.

Check:
$$7x = 12 + 6x$$
$$7(12) = 12 + 6(12)$$
$$84 = 12 + 72$$
$$84 = 84, \text{ true}$$

2e. Solve and check: $12 - 6x = 18 - 7x$

2f. Solve and check: $3x - 6 = 2x + 5$

$$3x - 6 = 2x + 5$$
$$3x - 2x - 6 = 2x - 2x + 5$$
$$x - 6 = 5$$
$$x - 6 + 6 = 5 + 6$$
$$x = 11$$

The solution set is $\{11\}$.

Check:
$$3x - 6 = 2x + 5$$
$$3(11) - 6 = 2(11) + 5$$
$$33 - 6 = 22 + 5$$
$$27 = 27, \text{ true}$$

2f. Solve and check: $4x + 2 = 3(x - 6) + 8$

Copyright © 2017 Pearson Education, Inc.

Learning Objective #3: Solve applied problems using formulas.

✔ Solved Problem #3

3. There is a relationship between the number of words in a child's vocabulary, V, and the child's age, A, in months, for ages between 15 and 50 months, inclusive.

   This relationship can be modeled by the formula
   $$V + 900 = 60A.$$

   Use the formula to find the number of words in a child's vocabulary at the age of 50 months.

   $$V + 900 = 60A$$
   $$V + 900 = 60(50)$$
   $$V + 900 = 3000$$
   $$V + 900 - 900 = 3000 - 900$$
   $$V = 2100$$

   At 50 months, a child will have a vocabulary of 2100 words.

✎ Pencil Problem #3 ✎

3. The cost, C, of an item (the price paid by a retailer) plus the markup, M, on that item (the retailer's profit) equals the selling price, S, of the item.

   This relationship is modeled by the formula
   $$C + M = S.$$

   For a particular computer, the selling price is $1850. If the markup is $150, find the cost to the retailer for the computer.

Answers for Pencil Problems *(Textbook Exercise references in parentheses)*:

1a. linear *(2.1 #1)*   **1b.** not linear *(2.1 #3)*   **1c.** not linear *(2.1 #5)*

2a. {23} *(2.1 #11)*   **2b.** {4} *(2.1 #19)*   **2c.** $\left\{-\dfrac{17}{12}\right\}$ *(2.1 #25)*

2d. {11} *(2.1 #45)*   **2e.** {6} *(2.1 #51)*   **2f.** {−12} *(2.1 #53)*

3. $1700 *(2.1 #63)*

Homework:

☐ **Review the Section 2.1 summary** on page 198 of the textbook.

☐ **Insert your homework** into this section of the *Learning Guide*. Show all work neatly and check your answers. Strive to work through difficulties when possible, making note of any exercises where you need additional help. Remember, even if your instructor assigns homework through *MyMathLab*, you should still write out your work.

Copyright © 2017 Pearson Education, Inc.

Section 2.2
The Multiplication Property of Equality

DO YOU FEEL SAFE????

You just heard some booming thunder shortly after you saw a huge flash of lightning!!!

How far away from you is that storm?

Well, one of the application exercises in this section of your textbook offers you a quick mathematical way to determine exactly that!

First Steps:

☐ **Take comprehensive notes** from your instructor's lecture and insert your notes into this section of the *Learning Guide*. Be sure to write down all examples, definitions, and other key concepts. Additional learning resources include the *Video Lecture Series*, the *PowerPoints*, and Section 2.2 of your textbook which begins on page 122.

☐ Complete the **Concept and Vocabulary Check** on page 129 of the textbook.

Guided Practice:

☐ Review each of the following *Solved Problems* and complete each *Pencil Problem*.

Learning Objective #1: Use the multiplication property of equality to solve equations.

✔ *Solved Problem #1*	✎ *Pencil Problem #1*✎
1a. Solve and check: $\dfrac{x}{3} = 12$	**1a.** Solve and check: $\dfrac{x}{6} = 5$

$$\frac{x}{3} = 12$$

$$3 \cdot \frac{x}{3} = 12 \cdot 3$$

$$1x = 36$$

$$x = 36$$

The solution set is $\{36\}$.

Check: $\dfrac{x}{3} = 12$

$$\frac{36}{3} = 12$$

$$12 = 12, \text{ true}$$

1b. Solve: $-11y = 44$

$-11y = 44$

$\dfrac{-11y}{-11} = \dfrac{44}{-11}$

$1x = -4$

$x = -4$

The solution set is $\{-4\}$.

1b. Solve: $-28 = 8z$

1c. Solve: $\dfrac{2}{3}y = 16$

$\dfrac{2}{3}y = 16$

$\dfrac{3}{2}\left(\dfrac{2}{3}y\right) = \dfrac{3}{2} \cdot 16$

$1y = 24$

$y = 24$

The solution set is $\{24\}$.

1c. Solve: $28 = -\dfrac{7}{2}x$

Learning Objective #2: Solve equations in the form $-x = c$.

✔ *Solved Problem #2*	✎ *Pencil Problem #2* ✎

2a. Solve: $-x = 5$

$-x = 5$

$-1x = 5$

$(-1)(-1x) = (-1)5$

$1x = -5$

$x = -5$

The solution set is $\{-5\}$.

2a. Solve: $-x = 17$

2b. Solve: $-x = -3$

$-x = -3$

$-1x = -3$

$(-1)(-1x) = (-1)(-3)$

$1x = 3$

$x = 3$

The solution set is $\{3\}$.

2b. Solve: $-47 = -y$

Copyright © 2017 Pearson Education, Inc.

Learning Objective #3: Use the addition and multiplication properties to solve equations.

✔ **Solved Problem #3**	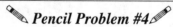 **Pencil Problem #3**
3a. Solve: $-4y - 15 = 25$	**3a.** Solve: $2x + 1 = 11$

$$-4y - 15 = 25$$
$$-4y - 15 + 15 = 25 + 15$$
$$-4y = 40$$
$$\frac{-4y}{-4} = \frac{40}{-4}$$
$$y = -10$$

The solution set is $\{-10\}$.

3b. Solve: $2x - 15 = -4x + 21$

3b. Solve: $6x + 14 = 2x - 2$

$$2x - 15 = -4x + 21$$
$$2x + 4x - 15 = -4x + 4x + 21$$
$$6x - 15 = 21$$
$$6x - 15 + 15 = 21 + 15$$
$$6x = 36$$
$$\frac{6x}{6} = \frac{36}{6}$$
$$x = 6$$

The solution set is $\{6\}$.

Learning Objective #4: Solve applied problems using formulas.

✔ **Solved Problem #4**

Pencil Problem #4

4. In 1980 the median weekly earnings for men with a bachelor's degree and higher was $427.

In 2013 the median weekly earnings for men with a bachelor's degree and higher was $1395.

Furthermore, the earnings for men with a bachelor's degree and higher can be described by the mathematical model.
$$M = 29n + 427,$$
where M represents median weekly earnings n years after 1980.

4. The Mach number is a measurement of speed, named after the man who suggested it, Ernst Mach (1838-1916). The formula
$$M = \frac{A}{740},$$
Indicates that the speed of an aircraft, A, in miles per hour, divided by the speed of sound, approximately 740 miles per hour, results in the Mach number, M.

Use the formula to determine the speed, in miles per hour, of the Concorde flying at Mach 2.03.

Copyright © 2017 Pearson Education, Inc.

4a. Does the formula underestimate or overestimate the median weekly earnings for men with a bachelor's degree and higher in 2013? By how much?

The median weekly earnings for men with a bachelor's degree and higher in 2013 was $1395. Since 2013 is 33 years after 1980, substitute 33 into the formula for n.

$M = 29n + 427$

$M = 29(33) + 427$

$M = 957 + 427$

$M = 1384$

The formula indicates that the median weekly earnings for men with a bachelor's degree and higher in 2013 was $1384. The formula underestimates the actual value of $1395 by $11.

4b. If trends shown by the formula continue, when will the median weekly earnings for men with a bachelor's degree and higher be $1442?

$$M = 29n + 427$$

$$1442 = 29n + 427$$

$$1442 - 427 = 29n + 427 - 427$$

$$1015 = 29n$$

$$\frac{1015}{29} = \frac{29n}{29}$$

$$35 = n$$

The formula estimates that 35 years after 1980, or in 2015, the median weekly earnings for men with a bachelor's degree and higher will be $1442.

Answers for Pencil Problems *(Textbook Exercise references in parentheses)*:

1a. {30}   *(2.2 #1)*   **1b.** $\left\{-\dfrac{7}{2}\right\}$ *(2.2 #9)*   **1c.** {−8}   *(2.2 #19)*   **2a.** {−17}   *(2.2 #21)*   **2b.** {47}   *(2.2 #23)*

3a. {5}   *(2.2 #29)*   **3b.** {−4}   *(2.2 #51)*   **4.** 1502.2 miles per hour   *(2.2 #69)*

Homework:

☐ **Review the Section 2.2 summary** on page 198 of the textbook.

☐ **Insert your homework** into this section of the *Learning Guide*. Show all work neatly and check your answers. Strive to work through difficulties when possible, making note of any exercises where you need additional help. Remember, even if your instructor assigns homework through *MyMathLab*, you should still write out your work.

   Copyright © 2017 Pearson Education, Inc.

Section 2.3
Solving Linear Equations

Slow Down or Pay the Fine!

In Massachusetts, speeding fines are determined by the mathematical formula
$$F = 10(x - 65) + 50,$$
where F is the cost, in dollars, of the fine if a person is caught driving x miles per hour.

In this section, you will learn to apply the formula to determine how fast a person was driving if you are told the amount of their fine.

First Steps:

☐ **Take comprehensive notes** from your instructor's lecture and insert your notes into this section of the *Learning Guide*. Be sure to write down all examples, definitions, and other key concepts. Additional learning resources include the *Video Lecture Series*, the *PowerPoints*, and Section 2.3 of your textbook which begins on page 132.

☐ Complete the **Concept and Vocabulary Check** on page 141 of the textbook.

Guided Practice:

☐ Review each of the following **Solved Problems** and complete each **Pencil Problem**.

Learning Objective #1: Solve linear equations.

✔ **Solved Problem #1**

1a. Solve: $-7x + 25 + 3x = 16 - 2x - 3$

Simplify the algebraic expression on each side.
$-7x + 25 + 3x = 16 - 2x - 3$
$\qquad -4x + 25 = 13 - 2x$

Collect variable terms on one side and constant terms on the other side.
$\qquad -4x + 25 = 13 - 2x$
$-4x + 25 + 2x = 13 - 2x + 2x$
$\qquad -2x + 25 = 13$
$-2x + 25 - 25 = 13 - 25$
$\qquad -2x = -12$

Isolate the variable and solve.
$$\frac{-2x}{-2} = \frac{-12}{-2}$$
$$x = 6$$

The solution set is $\{6\}$.

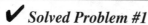 **Pencil Problem #1**

1a. Solve: $4x - 9x + 22 = 3x + 30$

1b. Solve: $4(2x+1)-29 = 3(2x-5)$

1b. Solve: $5(2x-8)-2 = 5(x-3)+3$

Simplify the algebraic expression on each side.
$$4(2x+1)-29 = 3(2x-5)$$
$$8x+4-29 = 6x-15$$
$$8x-25 = 6x-15$$

Collect variable terms on one side and constant terms on the other side.
$$8x-6x-25 = 6x-6x-15$$
$$2x-25 = -15$$
$$2x-25+25 = -15+25$$
$$2x = 10$$

Isolate the variable and solve.
$$\frac{2x}{2} = \frac{10}{2}$$
$$x = 5$$

The solution set is $\{5\}$.

Learning Objective #2: Solve linear equations containing fractions.

✔ Solved Problem #2

✎ Pencil Problem #2 ✎

2. Solve: $\dfrac{x}{4} = \dfrac{2x}{3} + \dfrac{5}{6}$

2. Solve: $\dfrac{y}{3} + \dfrac{2}{5} = \dfrac{y}{5} - \dfrac{2}{5}$

Begin by multiplying both sides of the equation by 12, the least common denominator.
$$\frac{x}{4} = \frac{2x}{3} + \frac{5}{6}$$
$$12 \cdot \frac{x}{4} = 12\left(\frac{2x}{3} + \frac{5}{6}\right)$$
$$12 \cdot \frac{x}{4} = 12 \cdot \frac{2x}{3} + 12 \cdot \frac{5}{6}$$
$$3x = 8x + 10$$
$$3x - 8x = 8x - 8x + 10$$
$$-5x = 10$$
$$\frac{-5x}{-5} = \frac{10}{-5}$$
$$x = -2$$

The solution set is $\{-2\}$.

Copyright © 2017 Pearson Education, Inc.

Learning Objective #3: Solve linear equations containing decimals.	
✔ **Solved Problem #3**	✎ **Pencil Problem #3**✎

3. Solve: $0.48x + 3 = 0.2(x - 6)$

First apply the distributive property to remove the parentheses, and then multiply both sides by 100 to clear the decimals.

$$0.48x + 3 = 0.2(x - 6)$$
$$0.48x + 3 = 0.2x - 1.2$$
$$100(0.48x + 3) = 100(0.2x - 1.2)$$
$$48x + 300 = 20x - 120$$
$$48x + 300 - 300 = 20x - 120 - 300$$
$$48x = 20x - 420$$
$$48x - 20x = 20x - 20x - 420$$
$$28x = -420$$
$$\frac{28x}{28} = \frac{-420}{28}$$
$$x = -15$$

The solution set is $\{-15\}$.

3. Solve: $0.3x - 4 = 0.1(x + 10)$

Learning Objective #4: Identify equations with no solution or infinitely many solutions.	
✔ **Solved Problem #4**	✎ **Pencil Problem #4**✎

4a. Solve: $3x + 7 = 3(x + 1)$

$$3x + 7 = 3(x + 1)$$
$$3x + 7 = 3x + 3$$
$$3x - 3x + 7 = 3x - 3x + 3$$
$$7 = 3$$

The original equation is equivalent to the false statement $7 = 3$. Thus, the equation has no solution.

The solution set is $\{ \ \}$.

4a. Solve: $4(x + 2) + 1 = 7x - 3(x - 2)$

4b. Solve: $3(x - 1) + 9 = 8x + 6 - 5x$

$$3(x - 1) + 9 = 8x + 6 - 5x$$
$$3x - 3 + 9 = 3x + 6$$
$$3x + 6 = 3x + 6$$
$$3x - 3x + 6 = 3x - 3x + 6$$
$$6 = 6$$

The original equation is equivalent to $6 = 6$, which is true for every value of x. The equation's solution is all real numbers or $\{x | x \text{ is a real number}\}$.

4b. Solve: $2(x + 4) = 4x + 5 - 2x + 3$

Copyright © 2017 Pearson Education, Inc.

Learning Objective #5: Solve applied problems using formulas.

✔ *Solved Problem #5*

5. It has been shown that persons with a low sense of humor have higher levels of depression in response to negative life events than those with a high sense of humor. This can be modeled by the following formulas:

Low-Humor Group: $D = \dfrac{10}{9}x + \dfrac{53}{9}$

High-Humor Group: $D = \dfrac{1}{9}x + \dfrac{26}{9}$

where x represents the intensity of a negative life event (from a low of 1 to a high of 10) and D is the level of depression in response to that event.

If the low-humor group averages a level of depression of 10 in response to a negative life event, what is the intensity of that event?

Low-Humor Group: $D = \dfrac{10}{9}x + \dfrac{53}{9}$

$$10 = \dfrac{10}{9}x + \dfrac{53}{9}$$

$$9 \cdot 10 = 9\left(\dfrac{10}{9}x + \dfrac{53}{9}\right)$$

$$90 = 10x + 53$$

$$90 - 53 = 10x + 53 - 53$$

$$37 = 10x$$

$$\dfrac{37}{10} = \dfrac{10x}{10}$$

$$3.7 = x$$

$$x = 3.7$$

The formula indicates that if the low-humor group averages a level of depression of 10 in response to a negative life event, the intensity of that event is 3.7.

✎ *Pencil Problem #5* ✎

5. The formula $p = 15 + \dfrac{5d}{11}$ describes the pressure of sea water, p, in pounds per square foot, at a depth of d feet below the surface.

The record depth for breath-held diving, by Francisco Ferreras (Cuba) off Grand Bahama Island, on November 14, 1993, involved pressure of 201 pounds per square foot. Use the formula to determine the depth to which Ferreras descended?

Answers for Pencil Problems *(Textbook Exercise references in parentheses)*:

1a. $\{-1\}$ *(2.3 #3)*   **1b.** $\{6\}$ *(2.3 #25)*   **2.** $\{-6\}$ *(2.3 #41)*   **3.** $\{25\}$ *(2.3 #51)*

4a. $\varnothing$ *(2.3 #67)*   **4b.** $\{x | x \text{ is a real number}\}$ *(2.3 #61)*   **5.** 409.2 feet *(2.3 #91)*

Homework:

☐ **Review the Section 2.3 summary** that begins on page 198 of the textbook.

☐ **Insert your homework** into this section of the *Learning Guide*. Show all work neatly and check your answers. Strive to work through difficulties when possible, making note of any exercises where you need additional help. Remember, even if your instructor assigns homework through *MyMathLab*, you should still write out your work.

  Copyright © 2017 Pearson Education, Inc.

What Is the Most Taboo Topic to Discuss at Work?

A survey asked about taboo topics to discuss at work. Common responses included... Religion, Politics, Money, Office Gossip, and Personal Life.

You will apply the techniques learned in this section of your textbook to determine the number of people that stated the most common response.

First Steps:

☐ **Take comprehensive notes** from your instructor's lecture and insert your notes into this section of the *Learning Guide*. Be sure to write down all examples, definitions, and other key concepts. Additional learning resources include the *Video Lecture Series*, the *PowerPoints*, and Section 2.4 of your textbook which begins on page 144.

☐ Complete the *Concept and Vocabulary Check* on page 152 of the textbook.

Guided Practice:

☐ Review each of the following *Solved Problems* and complete each *Pencil Problem*.

Learning Objective #1: Solve a formula for a variable.	
✔ *Solved Problem #1*	✎ *Pencil Problem #1* ✎

1a. Solve the formula $A = lw$ for l.

$A = lw$

$\dfrac{A}{w} = \dfrac{lw}{w}$

$\dfrac{A}{w} = l$

1a. Solve the formula $d = rt$ for r.

1b. Solve the formula $2l + 2w = P$ for l.

$2l + 2w = P$

$2l + 2w - 2w = P - 2w$

$2l = P - 2w$

$\dfrac{2l}{2} = \dfrac{P - 2w}{2}$

$l = \dfrac{P - 2w}{2}$

1b. Solve the formula $Ax + By = C$ for x.

Copyright © 2017 Pearson Education, Inc.

1c. Solve the formula $T = D + pm$ for m.

$$T = D + pm$$
$$T - D = pm$$
$$\frac{T - D}{p} = \frac{pm}{p}$$
$$\frac{T - D}{p} = m$$
$$m = \frac{T - D}{p}$$

1c. Solve the formula $y = mx + b$ for m.

1d. Solve the formula $\dfrac{x}{3} - 4y = 5$ for x.

$$\frac{x}{3} - 4y = 5$$
$$3\left(\frac{x}{3} - 4y\right) = 3 \cdot 5$$
$$3 \cdot \frac{x}{3} - 3 \cdot 4y = 3 \cdot 5$$
$$x - 12y = 15$$
$$x - 12y + 12y = 15 + 12y$$
$$x = 15 + 12y$$

1d. Solve the formula $\dfrac{c}{2} + 80 = 2F$ for c.

Learning Objective #2: Use the percent formula.

✔ **Solved Problem #2**

✎ **Pencil Problem #2** ✎

2a. What number is 9% of 50?

2a. What number is 3% of 200?

Use the formula $A = PB$: A is P percent of B.

$$\underset{A}{\boxed{\text{What}}} \ \underset{=}{\boxed{\text{is}}} \ \underset{0.09}{\boxed{9\%}} \ \underset{\cdot}{\boxed{\text{of}}} \ \underset{50}{\boxed{50?}}$$
$$A = 4.5$$

4.5 is 9% of 50.

Copyright © 2017 Pearson Education, Inc.

2b. 9 is 60% of what number?

Use the formula $A = PB$: A is P percent of B.

$$\boxed{9} \; \boxed{\text{is}} \; \boxed{60\%} \; \boxed{\text{of}} \; \boxed{\text{what?}}$$
$$9 = 0.60 \; \cdot \; B$$

$$\frac{9}{0.60} = \frac{0.60B}{0.60}$$

$$15 = B$$

9 is 60% of 15.

2b. 24% of what number is 40.8?

2c. 18 is what percent of 50?

Use the formula $A = PB$: A is P percent of B.

$$\boxed{18} \; \boxed{\text{is}} \; \boxed{\text{what percent}} \; \boxed{\text{of}} \; \boxed{50?}$$
$$18 = P \cdot 50$$

$$18 = P \cdot 50$$

$$\frac{18}{50} = \frac{50P}{50}$$

$$0.36 = P$$

To change 0.36 to a percent, move the decimal point two places to the right and add a percent sign.
$$0.36 = 36\%$$

18 is 36% of 50.

2c. 3 is what percent of 15?

Learning Objective #3: Solve applied problems involving percent change.

✔ Solved Problem #3

3a. A television regularly sells for $940. The sale price is $611.
Find the percent decrease in the television's price.

Use the formula $A = PB$: A is P percent of B.

Find the price decrease: $940 - $611 = $329

$$\boxed{\text{The price decrease}} \; \boxed{\text{is}} \; \boxed{\text{what percent}} \; \boxed{\text{of}} \; \boxed{\text{the original price?}}$$
$$329 = P \; \cdot \; 940$$

$$329 = P \cdot 940$$

$$\frac{329}{940} = \frac{940P}{940}$$

$$0.35 = P$$

To change 0.35 to a percent, move the decimal point two places to the right and add a percent sign. $0.35 = 35\%$

There was a 35% decrease.

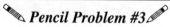 Pencil Problem #3

3a. Suppose that the local sales tax rate is 6% and you buy a car for $16,800.
How much tax is due?
What is the car's total cost?

3b. Suppose you paid $1200 in taxes. During year 1, taxes decrease by 20%. During year 2, taxes increase by 20%.
What do you pay in taxes for year 2?
How do your taxes for year 2 compare with what you originally paid, namely $1200?
If the taxes are not the same, find the percent increase or decrease.

First, find the amount that the taxes decreased from the original year to year 1: $0.20 \cdot \$1200 = \$240$
Next, subtract this amount of decrease from the original tax amount to obtain the amount paid in year 1.
Amount paid in year 1: $\$1200 - \$240 = \$960$

Now, find the amount that the taxes increased from year 1 to year 2: $0.20 \cdot \$960 = \$192$
Next, add this amount of increase to the amount paid in year 1 to obtain the amount paid in year 2.
Amount paid in year 2: $\$960 + \$192 = \$1152$

The taxes for year 2 are less than those originally paid.
Find the tax decrease: $\$1200 - \$1152 = \$48$

The tax decrease	is	what percent	of	the original tax?
48	=	P	$\cdot$	1200

$$48 = P \cdot 1200$$

$$\frac{48}{1200} = \frac{1200P}{1200}$$

$$0.04 = P$$

To change 0.04 to a percent, move the decimal point two places to the right and add a percent sign.
$0.04 = 4\%$

The overall tax decrease is 4%.

3b. Suppose that you put $10,000 in a rather risky investment recommended by your financial advisor. During the first year, your investment decreases by 30% of its original value. During the second year, your investment increases by 40% of its first-year value. Your advisor tells you that there must have been a 10% overall increase of your original $10,000 investment. Is your financial advisor using percentages properly? If not, what is the actual percent gain or loss on your original $10,000 investment?

Answers for Pencil Problems *(Textbook Exercise references in parentheses)*:

1a. $r = \dfrac{d}{t}$ *(2.4 #1)*   **1b.** $x = \dfrac{C - By}{A}$ *(2.4 #25)*   **1c.** $m = \dfrac{y - b}{x}$ *(2.4 #9)*   **1d.** $c = 4F - 160$ *(2.4 #17)*

2a. 6 *(2.4 #27)*   **2b.** 170 *(2.4 #33)*   **2c.** 20% *(2.4 #35)*

3a. tax due $1008; total cost $17,808 *(2.4 #65)*   **3b.** no; There is a 2% loss. *(2.4 #71)*

Homework:

☐ **Review the Section 2.4 summary** that begins on page 199 of the textbook.

☐ **Insert your homework** into this section of the *Learning Guide.* Show all work neatly and check your answers. Strive to work through difficulties when possible, making note of any exercises where you need additional help. Remember, even if your instructor assigns homework through *MyMathLab*, you should still write out your work.

Copyright © 2017 Pearson Education, Inc.

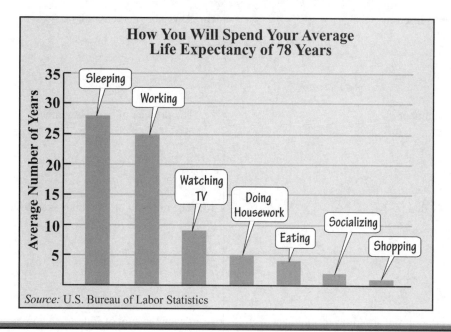

What are you doing with your life?

The bar graph shows the average number of years you will devote to seven of your most time-consuming activities.

In the Exercise Set of this section you will use problem solving techniques to take a closer look at how much time you sleep, watch TV, etc.

First Steps:

☐ **Take comprehensive notes** from your instructor's lecture and insert your notes into this section of the *Learning Guide*. Be sure to write down all examples, definitions, and other key concepts. Additional learning resources include the *Video Lecture Series*, the *PowerPoints*, and Section 2.5 of your textbook which begins on page 156.

☐ Complete the *Concept and Vocabulary Check* on page 165 of the textbook.

Guided Practice:

☐ Review each of the *Solved Problems* and complete each *Pencil Problem* on the following pages.

Learning Objective #1: Translate English phases into algebraic expressions.

✔ *Solved Problem #1*	✎ *Pencil Problem #1* ✎
For each of the following, let *x* represent the number. Use the given conditions to write an expression.	For each of the following, let *x* represent the number. Use the given conditions to write an expression.

1a. Five more than a number

$x + 5$

1a. A number increased by 60

1b. A number decreased by 5

$x - 5$

1b. A number decreased by 23

1c. Five times a number

$5x$

1c. The product of 7 and a number

1d. A number divided by 3

$\dfrac{x}{3}$

1d. The quotient of a number and 19

1e. Three times the sum of 1 and twice a number

$3(1 + 2x)$

1e. Twice the sum of four and a number

Achieving Success!

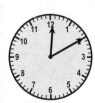

Do not expect to solve every word problem immediately. As you read each problem, underline the important parts. It's a good idea to read the problem at least twice.

Be persistent, but use the *"Ten Minutes of Frustration"* Rule. If you have exhausted every possible means for solving a problem and you are still bogged down, stop after ten minutes. Put a question mark by the exercise and move on. When you return to class, ask your professor for assistance.

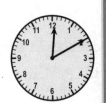

Copyright © 2017 Pearson Education, Inc.

Learning Objective #2: Solve algebraic word problems using linear equations.	
✔ *Solved Problem #2*	✎ *Pencil Problem #2*✐

2a. Four subtracted from six times a number is 68. Find the number.

Let x = the number.

$$6x - 4 = 68$$
$$6x - 4 + 4 = 68 + 4$$
$$6x = 72$$
$$x = 12$$

The number is 12.

2a. If the quotient of three times a number and five is increased by four, the result is 34. Find the number.

2b. Page numbers on facing pages of a book are consecutive integers. Two pages that face each other have 145 as the sum of their page numbers. What are the page numbers?

Let x = the page number of the first facing page.
Let $x + 1$ = the page number of the second facing page.

$$x + (x + 1) = 145$$
$$x + x + 1 = 145$$
$$2x + 1 = 145$$
$$2x + 1 - 1 = 145 - 1$$
$$2x = 144$$
$$x = 72$$
$$x + 1 = 73$$

The page numbers are 72 and 73.

2b. Page numbers on facing pages of a book are consecutive integers. Two pages that face each other have 629 as the sum of their page numbers. What are the page numbers?

2c. A taxi charges $2.00 to turn on the meter plus $0.25 for each eighth of a mile.
If you have $10.00, how many eighths of a mile can you go? How many miles is that?

Let x = the number of eighths of a mile traveled.

$$2 + 0.25x = 10$$
$$2 - 2 + 0.25x = 10 - 2$$
$$0.25x = 8$$
$$\frac{0.25x}{0.25} = \frac{8}{0.25}$$
$$x = 32$$

You can go 32 eighths of a mile.

That is equivalent to $\frac{32}{8} = 4$ miles.

2c. A car rental agency charges $200 per week plus $0.15 per mile to rent a car. How many miles can you travel in one week for $320?

Copyright © 2017 Pearson Education, Inc.

2d. After a 40% price reduction, an exercise machine sold for $564. What was the exercise machine's price before this reduction?

Let x = the original price.

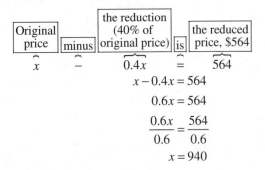

$$x - 0.4x = 564$$
$$0.6x = 564$$
$$\frac{0.6x}{0.6} = \frac{564}{0.6}$$
$$x = 940$$

The original price was $940.

2d. Including 6% sales tax, a car sold for $23,850. Find the price of the car before the tax was added.

Answers for Pencil Problems *(Textbook Exercise references in parentheses)*:

1a. $x + 60$ *(2.5 #1)*   **1b.** $x - 23$ *(2.5 #3)*   **1c.** $7x$ *(2.5 #5)*   **1d.** $\dfrac{x}{19}$ *(2.5 #7)*   **1e.** $2(x+4)$ *(2.5 #15)*

2a. $\dfrac{3x}{5} + 4 = 34$; 50 *(2.5 #19)*   **2b.** pages 314 and 315 *(2.5 #25)*   **2c.** 800 miles *(2.5 #29)*

2d. $22,500 *(2.5 #43)*

Homework:

☐ **Review the Section 2.5 summary** on page 200 of the textbook.

☐ **Insert your homework** into this section of the *Learning Guide*. Show all work neatly and check your answers. Strive to work through difficulties when possible, making note of any exercises where you need additional help. Remember, even if your instructor assigns homework through *MyMathLab*, you should still write out your work.

Copyright © 2017 Pearson Education, Inc.

Section 2.6
Problem Solving in Geometry

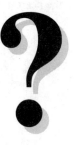 

Are they telling you the truth?

Did you know that graphs can be used to distort data, making it difficult for the viewer to learn the truth?

One potential source of misunderstanding involves geometric figures whose lengths are in the correct ratios for the displayed data, but whose areas or volumes are then varied to create a misimpression about how the data are changing over time.

Two such examples of misleading visual displays are given in the text and are related to the objectives of this section.

First Steps:

☐ **Take comprehensive notes** from your instructor's lecture and insert your notes into this section of the *Learning Guide*. Be sure to write down all examples, definitions, and other key concepts. Additional learning resources include the *Video Lecture Series*, the *PowerPoints*, and Section 2.6 of your textbook which begins on page 168.

☐ Complete the *Concept and Vocabulary Check* on page 176 of the textbook.

Guided Practice:

☐ Review each of the following *Solved Problems* and complete each *Pencil Problem*.

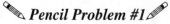

Learning Objective #1: Solve problems using formulas for perimeter and area.

✔ *Solved Problem #1*	✎ *Pencil Problem #1*
1. A sailboat has a triangular sail with an area of 24 square feet and a base that is 4 feet long. Find the height of the sail.	1. A triangle has a base of 5 feet and an area of 20 square feet. Find the triangle's height.

Use the formula $A = \frac{1}{2}bh$, where $A = 24$ and $b = 4$.

$A = \frac{1}{2}bh$

$24 = \frac{1}{2} \cdot 4 \cdot h$

$24 = 2h$

$12 = h$

The height of the sail is 12 ft.

Learning Objective #2: Solve problems using formulas for a circle's area and circumference.

✔ *Solved Problem #2*	✎ *Pencil Problem #2* ✎

2a. The diameter of a circular landing pad for helicopters is 40 feet. Find the area and circumference of the landing pad. Express answers in terms of π. Then round answers to the nearest square foot and foot, respectively.

Use the formulas for the area and circumference of a circle. The radius is 20 ft.

Area: $A = \pi r^2$

$\qquad A = \pi(20)^2$

$\qquad\quad = 400\pi$

$\qquad\quad \approx 1256 \ \text{ or } \ 1257$

The area is $400\pi \ \text{ft}^2$
or approximately 1256 ft^2 or 1257 ft^2.

Circumference: $C = 2\pi r$

$\qquad\qquad C = 2\pi(20)$

$\qquad\qquad\quad = 40\pi$

$\qquad\qquad\quad \approx 126$

The circumference is 40π ft or approximately 126 ft.

2a. The radius of a circle is 4 cm. Find the area and circumference of the circle. Express answers in terms of π. Then round answers to the nearest whole number.

2b. Which one of the following is the better buy: a large pizza with an 18-inch diameter for $20.00 or a medium pizza with a 14-inch diameter for $14.00?

The radius of the large pizza is 9 inches, and the radius of the medium pizza is 7 inches.

large pizza: $A = \pi r^2 = \pi(9 \ \text{in.})^2 = 81\pi \ \text{in.}^2 \approx 254 \ \text{in.}^2$

medium pizza: $A = \pi r^2 = \pi(7 \ \text{in.})^2 = 49\pi \ \text{in.}^2 \approx 154 \ \text{in.}^2$

For each pizza, find the price per square inch by dividing the price by the area.

Price per square inch for the large pizza:
$$\frac{\$20.00}{81\pi \ \text{in.}^2} \approx \frac{\$20.00}{254 \ \text{in.}^2} \approx \frac{\$0.08}{\text{in.}^2}$$

Price per square inch for the medium pizza:
$$\frac{\$14.00}{49\pi \ \text{in.}^2} \approx \frac{\$14.00}{154 \ \text{in.}^2} \approx \frac{\$0.09}{\text{in.}^2}.$$

The large pizza is the better buy.

2b. Which one of the following is the better buy: a large pizza with an 14-inch diameter for $12.00 or a medium pizza with a 7-inch diameter for $5.00?

     Copyright © 2017 Pearson Education, Inc.

Learning Objective #3: Solve problems using formulas for volume.

✔ **Solved Problem #3**	✎ *Pencil Problem #3*✎
3. A cylinder with a radius of 3 inches and a height of 5 inches has its height doubled. How many times greater is the volume of the larger cylinder than the volume of the smaller cylinder?	3. A cylinder with a radius of 3 inches and a height of 4 inches has its radius tripled. How many times greater is the volume of the larger cylinder than the volume of the smaller cylinder?

Smaller cylinder: $r = 3$ in., $h = 5$ in.

$V = \pi r^2 h$

$V = \pi(3)^2 \cdot 5$

$\quad = 45\pi$

The volume of the smaller cylinder is 45π in.^{3}.

Larger cylinder: $r = 3$ in., $h = 10$ in.

$V = \pi r^2 h$

$V = \pi(3)^2 \cdot 10$

$\quad = 90\pi$

The volume of the smaller cylinder is 90π in.^{3}.

The ratio of the volumes of the two cylinders is

$\dfrac{V_{\text{larger}}}{V_{\text{smaller}}} = \dfrac{90\pi \, \text{in.}^3}{45\pi \, \text{in.}^3} = \dfrac{2}{1}$.

Thus, the volume of the larger cylinder is 2 times the volume of the smaller cylinder.

Learning Objective #4: Solve problems involving the angles of a triangle.

✔ **Solved Problem #4**	✎ *Pencil Problem #4*✎
4. In a triangle, the measure of the first angle is three times the measure of the second angle. The measure of the third angle is $20°$ less than the second angle. What is the measure of each angle?	4. One angle of a triangle is twice as large as another. The measure of the third angle is $20°$ more than that of the smallest angle. What is the measure of each angle?

Let $3x =$ the measure of the first angle.
Let $x =$ the measure of the second angle.
Let $x - 20 =$ the measure of the third angle.

$3x + x + (x - 20) = 180$

$\qquad\qquad 5x - 20 = 180$

$\qquad\qquad\qquad 5x = 200$

$\qquad\qquad\qquad\quad x = 40$

$\qquad\qquad\qquad 3x = 120$

$\qquad\qquad x - 20 = 20$

The three angle measures are 120°, 40°, and 20°.

Learning Objective #5: Solve problems involving complementary and supplementary angles.

✔ *Solved Problem #5*	✎ *Pencil Problem #5* ✎
5. The measure of an angle is twice the measure of its complement. What is the angle's measure?	5. An angle's measure is $60°$ more than that of its complement. What is the angle's measure?

Step 1
Let x = the measure of the angle.

Step 2
Let $90 - x$ = the measure of its complement.

Step 3
The angle's measure is twice that of its complement, so the equation is $x = 2 \cdot (90 - x)$.

Step 4
Solve this equation
$$x = 2 \cdot (90 - x)$$
$$x = 180 - 2x$$
$$x + 2x = 180 - 2x + 2x$$
$$3x = 180$$
$$x = 60$$
The measure of the angle is $60°$.

Step 5
The complement of the angle is $90° - 60° = 30°$, and $60°$ is indeed twice $30°$.

Answers for Pencil Problems *(Textbook Exercise references in parentheses)*:

1. 8 feet *(2.6 #9)*

2a. Area is 16π cm^2 (approximately 50 cm^2) and circumference is 8π cm (approximately 25 cm). *(2.6 #13)*

2b. large pizza is better buy *(2.6 #59)*

3. 9 times *(2.6 #29)*

4. The three angle measures are $40°$, $80°$, and $60°$. *(2.6 #35)*   **5.** $75°$ *(2.6 #45)*

Homework:

☐ **Review the Section 2.6 summary** on page 201 of the textbook.

☐ **Insert your homework** into this section of the *Learning Guide*. Show all work neatly and check your answers. Strive to work through difficulties when possible, making note of any exercises where you need additional help. Remember, even if your instructor assigns homework through *MyMathLab*, you should still write out your work.

  Copyright © 2017 Pearson Education, Inc.

Section 2.7
Solving Linear Inequalities

YES, SPELLING COUNTS!

An online test of English spelling looked at how well people spelled difficult words.

Some of the words that appeared on the test include:
weird, cemetery, accommodation, harass, supersede, and inoculate.
(How well would you have done?)

We will apply the concept of linear inequalities to compare and contrast the success rates of spelling these difficult words.

First Steps:

☐ **Take comprehensive notes** from your instructor's lecture and insert your notes into this section of the *Learning Guide*. Be sure to write down all examples, definitions, and other key concepts. Additional learning resources include the *Video Lecture Series*, the *PowerPoints*, and Section 2.7 of your textbook which begins on page 182.

☐ Complete the *Concept and Vocabulary Check* on page 194 of the textbook.

Guided Practice:

☐ Review each of the following *Solved Problems* and complete each *Pencil Problem*.

Learning Objective #1: Graph the solutions of an inequality on a number line.

✔ *Solved Problem #1*	✎ *Pencil Problem #1*✎
1a. Graph the solution of the inequality: $x < 4$	**1a.** Graph the solution of the inequality: $x > 5$
The solutions of $x < 4$ are all real numbers that are less than 4. They are graphed on a number line by shading all points to the left of 4. The parenthesis at 4 indicates that 4 is not a solution. The arrow shows that the graph extends indefinitely to the left. 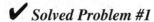	
1b. Graph the solution of the inequality: $-4 \le x < 1$	**1b.** Graph the solution of the inequality: $-2 < x \le 6$
The solutions of $-4 \le x < 1$ are all real numbers between -4 and 1, not including 1 but including -4. The square bracket at -4 shows that -4 is a solution. The parenthesis at 1 indicates that 1 is not a solution. Shading indicates the other solutions. 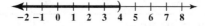	

Copyright © 2017 Pearson Education, Inc.

Learning Objective #2: Use interval notation.

✔ **Solved Problem #2**	✎ **Pencil Problem #2**✎
2a. Express the solution set of the inequality in interval notation and graph the interval: $x \geq 0$	**2a.** Express the solution set of the inequality in interval notation and graph the interval: $x \leq 3$

The solutions of $x \geq 0$ are all real numbers greater than or equal to 0.
Use a square bracket at 0 because 0 is a solution.
Since the solution extends indefinitely to the right, use a parenthesis at ∞.

$[0, \infty)$

Graph:

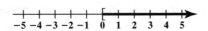

2b. Express the solution set of the inequality in interval notation and graph the interval: $x < 5$

The solutions of $x < 5$ are all real numbers less than 5.
Since the solution extends indefinitely to the left, use a parenthesis at $-\infty$.
Use a parenthesis at 5 because 5 is not a solution.

$(-\infty, 5)$

Graph:

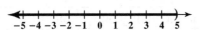

2b. Express the solution set of the inequality in

interval notation and graph the interval: $x > \dfrac{5}{2}$

Learning Objective #3: Understand properties used to solve linear inequalities.

✔ **Solved Problem #3**	✎ **Pencil Problem #3**✎
3. *True* or *False*: When we add (or subtract) a negative number to (or from) both sides of an inequality, the direction of the inequality symbol is reversed.	**3.** *True* or *False*: When we multiply or divide both sides of an inequality by a negative number, the direction of the inequality symbol is reversed.

False; This rule applies to multiplication and division.

Learning Objective #4: Solve linear inequalities.

✔ **Solved Problem #4**	✎ **Pencil Problem #4**✎
4a. Solve: $x + 6 < 9$	**4a.** Solve: $x - 3 > 4$

$x + 6 < 9$
$x + 6 - 6 < 9 - 6$
$x < 3$

The solution set is $(-\infty, 3)$ or $\{x | x < 3\}$.

Copyright © 2017 Pearson Education, Inc.

4b. Solve: $\dfrac{1}{4}x < 2$

$$\dfrac{1}{4}x < 2$$

$$4 \cdot \dfrac{1}{4}x < 4 \cdot 2$$

$$x < 8$$

The solution set is $(-\infty, 8)$ or $\{x \mid x < 8\}$.

4b. Solve: $-4y \le \dfrac{1}{2}$

4c. Solve: $-6x < 18$

$$-6x < 18$$

$$\dfrac{-6x}{-6} > \dfrac{18}{-6}$$

$$x > -3$$

The solution set is $(-3, \infty)$ or $\{x \mid x > -3\}$.

4c. Solve: $4x < 20$

Learning Objective #5: Identify inequalities with no solution or true for all real numbers.

✔ *Solved Problem #5*

✎ *Pencil Problem #5* ✐

5a. Solve: $4(x+2) > 4x + 15$

$$4(x+2) > 4x + 15$$

$$4x + 8 > 4x + 15$$

$$4x - 4x + 8 > 4x - 4x + 15$$

$$8 > 15, \text{ false}$$

There is no solution or $\{\ \}$.

5a. Solve: $4x - 4 < 4(x - 5)$

5b. Solve: $3(x+1) \ge 2x + 1 + x$

$$3(x+1) \ge 2x + 1 + x$$

$$3x + 3 \ge 3x + 1$$

$$3x - 3x + 3 \ge 3x - 3x + 1$$

$$3 \ge 1, \text{ true}$$

The solution is $(-\infty, \infty)$ or $\{x \mid x \text{ is a real number}\}$.

5b. Solve: $2(x+3) > 2x + 1$

Copyright © 2017 Pearson Education, Inc.

Learning Objective #6: Solve problems using linear inequalities.

✔ *Solved Problem #6*	✎ *Pencil Problem #6*✎
6. To earn a B in a course, you must have a final average of at least 80%. On the first three examinations, you have grades of 82%, 74%, and 78%. If the final examination counts as two grades, what must you get on the final to earn a B in the course?	**6.** An elevator at a construction site has a maximum capacity of 3000 pounds. If the elevator operator weighs 245 pounds and each cement bag weighs 95 pounds, how many bags of cement can be safely lifted on the elevator in one trip?

Let x = your grade on the final examination.

$$\frac{82+74+78+x+x}{5} \geq 80$$

$$\frac{234+2x}{5} \geq 80$$

$$5\left(\frac{234+2x}{5}\right) \geq 5 \cdot 80$$

$$234+2x \geq 400$$

$$234-234+2x \geq 400-234$$

$$2x \geq 166$$

$$x \geq 83$$

To earn a B you must get at least an 83% on the final examination.

Answers for Pencil Problems *(Textbook Exercise references in parentheses)*:

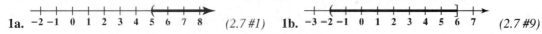

1a. *(2.7 #1)*   **1b.** *(2.7 #9)*

2a. $(-\infty, 3]$ *(2.7 #13)*   **2b.** $\left(\frac{5}{2}, \infty\right)$ *(2.7 #15)*

3. True *(2.7 #45,47)*

4a. $(7, \infty)$ *(2.7 #21)*   **4b.** $\left[-\frac{1}{8}, \infty\right)$ *(2.7 #53)*   **4c.** $(-\infty, 5)$ *(2.7 #43)*

5a. There is no solution or $\{\ \}$. *(2.7 #81)*   **5b.** The solution is $(-\infty, \infty)$ or $\{x | x \text{ is a real number}\}$. *(2.7 #87)*

6. up to 29 bags of cement *(2.7 #111)*

Homework:

☐ **Review the Section 2.7 summary** that begins on page 201 of the textbook.

☐ **Insert your homework** into this section of the *Learning Guide*. Show all work neatly and check your answers. Strive to work through difficulties when possible, making note of any exercises where you need additional help. Remember, even if your instructor assigns homework through *MyMathLab*, you should still write out your work.

        Copyright © 2017 Pearson Education, Inc.

One of the best ways to learn how to solve a word problem in algebra is to design word problems of your own. Creating a word problem makes you very aware of precisely how much information is needed to solve the problem. You must also focus on the best way to present information to a reader and on how much information to give. As you write your problem, you gain skills that will help you solve problems created by others.

The group should design five different word problems that can be solved using an algebraic equation. All of the problems should be on different topics. For example, the group should not have more than one problem on finding a number. The group should turn in both the problems and their algebraic solutions.

Copyright © 2017 Pearson Education, Inc.

Getting Ready for the Chapter 2 Test

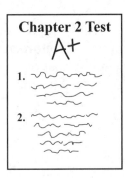

Chapter 2 Test

One of the best ways to prepare for a test is to stay on top of your studying, keeping up as your professor proceeds from section to section. Falling behind on one section often makes it difficult to understand the material in the following section. Never wait until the last minute to study for an exam.

Below are several actions that will help you stay organized as you prepare for your test.

How to prepare for your Chapter Test:

☐ **Write down any details that your instructor shares about the test.**
In addition to items such as location, date, time, and essentials to bring, be sure to listen carefully for specific information about the topics covered. Communicate with your instructor concerning any details that may be unclear to you.

☐ **Read the Chapter Summary that begins on page 198 of your textbook.**
Study the appropriate sections in the Chapter Summary. This summary contains the most important material in each section including, definitions, concepts, procedures, and examples.

☐ **Review your *Learning Guide.***
Go back through the *Solved Problems* and *Pencil Problems* in this chapter of your *Learning Guide*. You may find it helpful to cover up solutions and work through the problems again.

☐ **Study your notes and homework.**
Read through your class notes that you took during this unit, and review the corresponding homework assignments.

☐ **Review quizzes and other feedback from your professor.**
Review any quizzes you have taken and be sure you understand any errors that you made. Seek help with any concepts that are still unclear.

☐ **Complete the Review Exercises that begin on page 203 of your textbook.**
Work the assigned problems from the Review Exercises. These exercises represent the most significant problems for each of the chapter's sections. The answers for all Review Exercises are in the back of your textbook.

☐ **Take the Chapter Test that begins on page 206 of your textbook.**
- Find a quiet place to take the Chapter Test.
- Do not use notes, index cards, or any resources other than those your instructor will allow during the actual test.
- After completing the entire test, check your answers in the back of the textbook.
- Watch the *Chapter Test Prep Video* to review any exercises you may have missed.

Copyright © 2017 Pearson Education, Inc.

Chapter 3.R Linear Equations and Inequalities in Two Variables
Integrated Review

Learning Objectives
1. Evaluate algebraic expressions.v
2. Determine whether a number is a solution of an equation.

Learning Objective #1: Evaluate algebraic expressions.

✔ *Solved Problem #1*	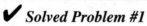 *Pencil Problem #1*
1a. Evaluate $6 + 2x$ for $x = 10$.	**1a.** Evaluate $2(x + 5)$ for $x = 4$.

$$6 + 2x = 6 + 2(10)$$
$$= 6 + 20$$
$$= 26$$

1b. Evaluate $\dfrac{6x - y}{2y - x - 8}$ for $x = 3$ and $y = 8$.

1b. Evaluate $\dfrac{21}{x} + \dfrac{35}{y}$ for $x = 7$ and $y = 5$.

$$\dfrac{6x - y}{2y - x - 8} = \dfrac{6(3) - 8}{2(8) - 3 - 8}$$
$$= \dfrac{18 - 8}{16 - 3 - 8}$$
$$= \dfrac{10}{5}$$
$$= 2$$

Learning Objective #2: Determine whether a number is a solution of an equation.

✔ *Solved Problem #2*	✎ *Pencil Problem #2* ✎

2a. Determine whether 6 is a solution of the equation.

$$9x - 3 = 42$$

To determine whether 6 is a solution, substitute 6 for x.

$$9x - 3 = 42$$
$$9(6) - 3 = 42$$
$$54 - 3 = 42$$
$$51 \neq 42$$

Because the values on both sides of the equation are not the same, the number 6 is not a solution of the equation.

2a. Determine whether 20 is a solution of the equation.

$$30 - y = 10$$

2b. Determine whether 3 is a solution of the equation.

$$2(y + 3) = 5y - 3$$

To determine whether 3 is a solution, substitute 3 for y.

$$2(y + 3) = 5y - 3$$
$$2(3 + 3) = 5(3) - 3$$
$$2(6) = 15 - 3$$
$$12 = 12$$

Because the values on both sides of the equation are the same, the number 3 is a solution of the equation.

2b. Determine whether 7 is a solution of the equation.

$$2(w + 1) = 3(w - 1)$$

Answers for Pencil Problems:

1a. 18   **1b.** 10   **2a.** solution   **2b.** not a solution

Copyright © 2017 Pearson Education, Inc.

Section 3.1
Graphing Linear Equations in Two Variables

Throw me the BALL!

From the time a football leaves a quarterback's hand until it is caught by the receiver, it follows a predictable path.

The Exercise Set of this section of the textbook will show how a graph can be used to analyze the position of the football during its flight.

First Steps:

☐ **Take comprehensive notes** from your instructor's lecture and insert your notes into this section of the *Learning Guide*. Be sure to write down all examples, definitions, and other key concepts. Additional learning resources include the *Video Lecture Series*, the *PowerPoints*, and Section 3.1 of your textbook which begins on page 209.

☐ Complete the *Concept and Vocabulary Check* on page 219 of the textbook.

Guided Practice:

☐ Review each of the following *Solved Problems* and complete each *Pencil Problem*.

Learning Objective #1: Plot ordered pairs in the rectangular coordinate system.

✔ *Solved Problem #1*	✎ *Pencil Problem #1* ✎

1. Plot the points:
    $A(-2, 4)$, $B(4, -2)$, $C(-3, 0)$, and $D(0, -3)$.
	1. Plot the points:
	    $A(3, 5)$, $B(-5, 1)$, $C(-3, -1)$.

From the origin, point *A* is left 2 units and up 4 units.

From the origin, point *B* is right 4 units and down 2 units.

From the origin, point *C* is left 3 units.

From the origin, point *D* is down 3 units.

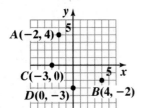

Copyright © 2017 Pearson Education, Inc.

Learning Objective #2: Find coordinates of points in the rectangular coordinate system.

✔ **Solved Problem #2**	✎ *Pencil Problem #2* ✎

2. Determine the coordinates of points E, F, and G.

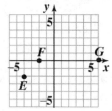

2. Determine the coordinates of points A, C, and E.

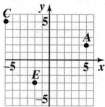

From the origin, point E is left 4 units and down 2 units.
Coordinates: $E(-4,-2)$

From the origin, point F is left 2 units.
Coordinates: $F(-2,0)$

From the origin, point G is right 6 units.
Coordinates: $G(6,0)$

Learning Objective #3: Determine whether an ordered pair is a solution of an equation.

✔ **Solved Problem #3**	✎ *Pencil Problem #3* ✎

3a. Determine whether the ordered pair $(3,-2)$ is a solution of the equation $x-3y=9$.

$$x-3y=9$$
$$3-3(-2)=9$$
$$3+6=9$$
$$9=9, \text{ true}$$

$(3,-2)$ is a solution.

3a. Determine whether the ordered pair $(0,6)$ is a solution of the equation $y=2x+6$.

3b. Determine whether the ordered pair $(-2,3)$ is a solution of the equation $x-3y=9$.

$$x-3y=9$$
$$-2-3(3)=9$$
$$-2-9=9$$
$$-11=9, \text{ false}$$

$(-2,3)$ is not a solution.

3b. Determine whether the ordered pair $(2,-2)$ is a solution of the equation $y=2x+6$.

Copyright © 2017 Pearson Education, Inc.

Learning Objective #4: Find solutions of an equation in two variables.

✔ Solved Problem #4

4. Find five solutions of $y = 3x + 2$.

Select integers for x, starting with –2 and ending with 2.

x	$y = 3x + 2$	(x, y)
–2	$y = 3(-2) + 2$ $= -6 + 2$ $= -4$	$(-2, -4)$
–1	$y = 3(-1) + 2$ $= -3 + 2$ $= -1$	$(-1, -1)$
0	$y = 3(0) + 2$ $= 0 + 2$ $= 2$	$(0, 2)$
1	$y = 3(1) + 2$ $= 3 + 2$ $= 5$	$(1, 5)$
2	$y = 3(2) + 2$ $= 6 + 2$ $= 8$	$(2, 8)$

✎ Pencil Problem #4 ✎

4. Find five solutions of $y = -3x + 7$.

Select integers for x, starting with –2 and ending with 2.

Learning Objective #5: Use point plotting to graph linear equations.

✔ Solved Problem #5

5a. Graph the equation: $y = 2x$

First, make a table of values:

x	$y = 2x$	(x, y)
–2	$y = 2(-2) = -4$	$(-2, -4)$
–1	$y = 2(-1) = -2$	$(-1, -2)$
0	$y = 2(0) = 0$	$(0, 0)$
1	$y = 2(1) = 2$	$(1, 2)$
2	$y = 2(2) = 4$	$(2, 4)$

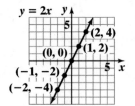

✎ Pencil Problem #5 ✎

5a. Graph the equation: $y = x$

Copyright © 2017 Pearson Education, Inc.

5b. Graph the equation: $y = \frac{1}{2}x + 2$

First, make a table of values:

x	$y = \frac{1}{2}x + 2$	(x, y)
-4	$y = \frac{1}{2}(-4) + 2 = 0$	$(-4, 0)$
-2	$y = \frac{1}{2}(-2) + 2 = 1$	$(-2, 1)$
0	$y = \frac{1}{2}(0) + 2 = 2$	$(0, 2)$
2	$y = \frac{1}{2}(2) + 2 = 3$	$(2, 3)$
4	$y = \frac{1}{2}(4) + 2 = 4$	$(4, 4)$

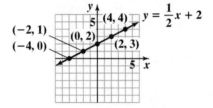

5b. Graph the equation: $y = -\frac{3}{2}x + 1$

Learning Objective #6: Use graphs of linear equations to solve problems.

✔ **Solved Problem #6**

6. The mathematical model $D = 1.4n + 1$ describes the percentage of consumers, D, who paid primarily with debit cards n years after 1995.

6a. Let $n = 0, 5, 10,$ and 15. Make a table of values showing four solutions of the equation.

n	$D = 1.4n + 1$	(n, D)
0	$D = 1.4(0) + 1$ $= 0 + 1$ $= 1$	$(0, 1)$
5	$D = 1.4(5) + 1$ $= 7 + 1$ $= 8$	$(5, 8)$
10	$D = 1.4(10) + 1$ $= 14 + 1$ $= 15$	$(10, 15)$
15	$D = 1.4(15) + 1$ $= 21 + 1$ $= 22$	$(15, 22)$

✎ **Pencil Problem #6** ✎

6. For the period from 2000 through 2010, the percentage viewing a college Education as essential for success increased on average by approximately 2.4 each year. These conditions can be described by the mathematical model $S = 2.4n + 31$, where S is the percentage of U.S. adults who viewed college as essential for success n years after 2000.

6a. Let $n = 0, 5, 10, 15$ and 20. Make a table of values showing five solutions of the equation.

Copyright © 2017 Pearson Education, Inc.

6b. Graph the formula in a rectangular coordinate system.

Plot the points from the table of values. Then use a straightedge to draw the line though them.

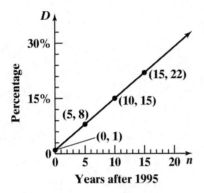

6c. Use your graph from part (b) to estimate the percentage of consumers who will pay primarily with debit cards in 2015.

According to the graph, about 29% of consumers will pay primarily with debit cards in 2015.

6d. Use the formula to project the percentage of consumers who will pay primarily by debit cards in 2015.

2015 is 20 years after 1995. Therefore, substitute 20 into the formula for n.

$D = 1.4n + 1$
$D = 1.4(20) + 1$
$\quad = 28 + 1$
$\quad = 29$

According to the formula, about 29% of consumers will pay primarily with debit cards in 2015.

6b. Graph the formula in a rectangular coordinate system.
Suggestion: Let each tick mark on the horizontal axis, labeled n, represent 5 units. Extend the horizontal axis to include $n = 25$. Let each tick mark on the vertical axis, labeled S, represent 10 units and extend the axis to include $S = 100$.

6c. Use your graph from part (b) to estimate the percentage of U.S. adults who will view college as essential for success in 2018.

6d. Use the formula to project the percentage of U.S. adults who will view college as essential for success in 2018.

Answers for Pencil Problems *(Textbook Exercise references in parentheses)*:

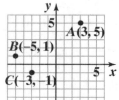

1. *(3.1 #1, #3, and #5)*

2. *A* (5,2), *C* (−6,5), *E*(−2,−3) *(3.1 #25, #27, and # 29)*

3a. (0,6) is a solution *(3.1 #41)* **3b.** (2,−2) is not a solution *(3.1 #41)*

x	$y = -3x + 7$	(x, y)
−2	$y = -3(-2) + 7 = 13$	$(-2, 13)$
−1	$y = -3(-1) + 7 = 10$	$(-1, 10)$
0	$y = -3(0) + 7 = 7$	$(0, 7)$
1	$y = -3(1) + 7 = 4$	$(1, 4)$
4. 2	$y = -3(2) + 7 = 1$	$(2, 1)$

(3.1 #55)

5a. 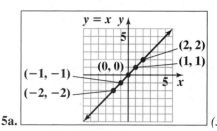 *(3.1 #57)* **5b.** 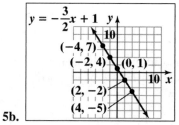 *(3.1 #73)*

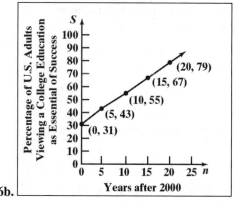

n	$S = 2.4n + 31$	(n, S)
0	$S = 2.4(0) + 31 = 31$	$(0, 31)$
5	$S = 2.4(5) + 31 = 43$	$(5, 43)$
10	$S = 2.4(10) + 31 = 55$	$(10, 55)$
15	$S = 2.4(15) + 31 = 67$	$(15, 67)$
6a. 20	$S = 2.4(20) + 31 = 79$	$(20, 79)$

(3.1 #93a) **6b.** *(3.1 #93b)*

6c. approximately 74% *(3.1 #93c)* **6d.** 74.2% *(3.1 #93d)*

Homework:

☐ **Review the Section 3.1 summary** on page 272 of the textbook.

☐ **Insert your homework** into this section of the *Learning Guide*. Show all work neatly and check your answers. Strive to work through difficulties when possible, making note of any exercises where you need additional help. Remember, even if your instructor assigns homework through *MyMathLab*, you should still write out your work.

Copyright © 2017 Pearson Education, Inc.

Section 3.2
Graphing Linear Equations Using Intercepts

It's all downhill from here!!!!

It seems that the value of a new car drops drastically the moment that you drive it off the lot!

This section of your textbook contains exercises that use mathematical models to explore the depreciation of automobiles.

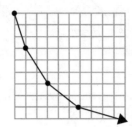

First Steps:

☐ **Take comprehensive notes** from your instructor's lecture and insert your notes into this section of the *Learning Guide*. Be sure to write down all examples, definitions, and other key concepts. Additional learning resources include the *Video Lecture Series*, the *PowerPoints*, and Section 3.2 of your textbook which begins on page 223.

☐ Complete the *Concept and Vocabulary Check* on page 231 of the textbook.

Guided Practice:

☐ Review each of the following *Solved Problems* and complete each *Pencil Problem*.

Learning Objective #1: Use a graph to identify intercepts.

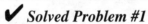

✔ *Solved Problem #1*	✎ *Pencil Problem #1* ✎
1a. Identify the *x*- and *y*- intercepts:	**1a.** Identify the *x*- and *y*- intercepts:

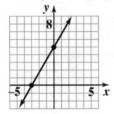

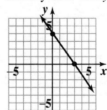

The graph crosses the *x*-axis at (–3,0).
Thus, the *x*-intercept is –3.

The graph crosses the *y*-axis at (0,5).
Thus, the *y*-intercept is 5.

1b. Identify the x- and y- intercepts:

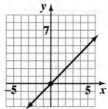

The graph crosses the x-axis at (0,0).
Thus, the x-intercept is 0.

The graph crosses the y-axis at (0,0).
Thus, the y-intercept is 0.

1b. Identify the x- and y- intercepts:

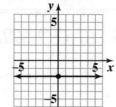

Learning Objective #2: Graph a linear equation in two variables using intercepts.

✔ *Solved Problem #2*

2a. Find the x-intercept of the graph of $4x - 3y = 12$.

To find the x-intercept, let $y = 0$ and solve for x.

$$4x - 3y = 12$$
$$4x - 3(0) = 12$$
$$4x = 12$$
$$x = 3$$

The x-intercept is 3.

✎ *Pencil Problem #2*✎

2a. Find the x-intercept of the graph of $2x + 5y = 20$.

2b. Find the y-intercept of the graph of $4x - 3y = 12$.

To find the y-intercept, let $x = 0$ and solve for y.

$$4x - 3y = 12$$
$$4(0) - 3y = 12$$
$$-3y = 12$$
$$y = -4$$

The y-intercept is –4.

2b. Find the y-intercept of the graph of $2x + 5y = 20$.

Copyright © 2017 Pearson Education, Inc.

2c. Use intercepts to graph $2x+3y=6$.

Find the x-intercept.
Let $y=0$ and solve for x.
$$2x+3y=6$$
$$2x+3(0)=6$$
$$2x=6$$
$$x=3$$
The x-intercept is 3.

Find the y-intercept.
Let $x=0$ and solve for y.
$$2x+3y=6$$
$$2(0)+3y=6$$
$$3y=6$$
$$y=2$$
The y-intercept is 2.

Find a checkpoint.
For example, let $x=1$ and solve for y.
$$2x+3y=6$$
$$2(1)+3y=6$$
$$2+3y=6$$
$$3y=4$$
$$y=\frac{4}{3} \text{ or } 1\frac{1}{3}$$

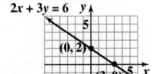

2c. Use intercepts to graph $6x-9y=18$.

Copyright © 2017 Pearson Education, Inc.

2d. Graph: $x + 3y = 0$

2d. Graph: $x + 2y = 0$

Because the constant on the right is 0, the graph passes through the origin. The *x*- and *y*-intercepts are both 0. Thus, we will need to find two more points.

Let $y = -1$ and solve for *x*.

$$x + 3y = 0$$
$$x + 3(-1) = 0$$
$$x - 3 = 0$$
$$x = 3$$

Let $y = 1$ and solve for *x*.

$$x + 3y = 0$$
$$x + 3(1) = 0$$
$$x + 3 = 0$$
$$x = -3$$

Use these three solutions of (0,0), (3,–1), and (–3,1).

$x + 3y = 0$

Copyright © 2017 Pearson Education, Inc.

Learning Objective #3: Graph horizontal or vertical lines.

✔ *Solved Problem #3*

3a. Graph: $y = 3$

As demonstrated in the table below, all ordered pairs that are solutions of $y = 3$ have a value of y that is always 3.

x	$y = 3$	(x, y)
-2	3	$(-2, 3)$
0	3	$(0, 3)$
1	3	$(1, 3)$

Thus the line is horizontal.

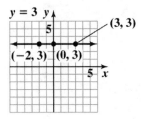

3b. Graph: $x = -2$

As demonstrated in the table below, all ordered pairs that are solutions of $x = -2$ have a value of x that is always -2.

$x = -2$	y	(x, y)
-2	3	$(-2, 3)$
-2	0	$(-2, 0)$
-2	-2	$(-2, -2)$

Thus the line is vertical.

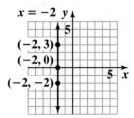

✎ *Pencil Problem #3* ✎

3a. Graph: $y = -2$

3b. Graph: $x = 2$

Answers for Pencil Problems *(Textbook Exercise references in parentheses)*:

1a. *x*-intercept is 3 and *y*-intercept is 4 *(3.2 #1)*

1b. no *x*-intercept and *y*-intercept is −2 *(3.2 #7)*

2a. *x*-intercept is 10 *(3.2 #9)*

2b. *y*-intercept is 4 *(3.2 #9)*

2c. 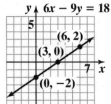 *(3.2 #23)*

2d. 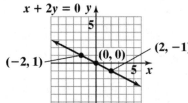 *(3.2 #35)*

3a. 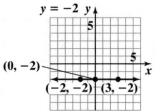 *(3.2 #49)*

3b. 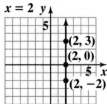 *(3.2 #51)*

Homework:

☐ **Review the Section 3.2 summary** that begins on page 272 of the textbook.

☐ **Insert your homework** into this section of the *Learning Guide*. Show all work neatly and check your answers. Strive to work through difficulties when possible, making note of any exercises where you need additional help. Remember, even if your instructor assigns homework through *MyMathLab*, you should still write out your work.

     Copyright © 2017 Pearson Education, Inc.

Are You Stressed Out?

If you are, you might be happy to learn that as we age, daily stress and worry decrease, but happiness increases!

For example, 49% of 22-year-olds reported having "a lot of stress," but only 29% of 62-year olds reported the same high stress level.

An application exercise in this section will utilize the concept of slope to mathematically analyze this research.

First Steps:

☐ **Take comprehensive notes** from your instructor's lecture and insert your notes into this section of the *Learning Guide*. Be sure to write down all examples, definitions, and other key concepts. Additional learning resources include the *Video Lecture Series*, the *PowerPoints*, and Section 3.3 of your textbook which begins on page 234.

☐ Complete the *Concept and Vocabulary Check* on page 241 of the textbook.

Guided Practice:

☐ Review each of the following *Solved Problems* and complete each *Pencil Problem*.

Learning Objective #1: Compute a line's slope.	
✔ *Solved Problem #1*	✎ *Pencil Problem #1*✎

1a. Find the slope of the line passing through the pair of points: $(4, -2)$ and $(-1, 5)$.

Let $(x_1, y_1) = (4, -2)$ and $(x_2, y_2) = (-1, 5)$.

$$m = \frac{\text{Change in } y}{\text{Change in } x} = \frac{y_2 - y_1}{x_2 - x_1} = \frac{5 - (-2)}{-1 - 4} = \frac{7}{-5} = -\frac{7}{5}$$

The slope is $-\dfrac{7}{5}$.

Since the slope is negative, the line falls from left to right.

1a. Find the slope of the line passing through the pair of points: $(4, 7)$ and $(8, 10)$.

Copyright © 2017 Pearson Education, Inc.

1b. Find the slope of the line passing through $(6,5)$ and $(2,5)$ or state that the slope is undefined. Indicate if the line is horizontal or vertical.

Let $(x_1, y_1) = (6,5)$ and $(x_2, y_2) = (2,5)$.

$$m = \frac{\text{Change in } y}{\text{Change in } x} = \frac{y_2 - y_1}{x_2 - x_1}$$
$$= \frac{5-5}{2-6}$$
$$= \frac{0}{-4}$$
$$= 0$$

Since the slope is 0, the line is horizontal.

1b. Find the slope of the line passing through $(4,-2)$ and $(3,-2)$ or state that the slope is undefined.
Indicate if the line is horizontal or vertical.

1c. Find the slope of the line passing through $(1,6)$ and $(1,4)$ or state that the slope is undefined. Indicate if the line is horizontal or vertical.

Let $(x_1, y_1) = (1,6)$ and $(x_2, y_2) = (1,4)$.

$$m = \frac{\text{Change in } y}{\text{Change in } x} = \frac{y_2 - y_1}{x_2 - x_1}$$
$$= \frac{4-6}{1-1}$$
$$= \frac{-2}{0}$$

Because division by 0 is undefined the slope is undefined.

Since the slope is undefined, the line is vertical.

1c. Find the slope of the line passing through $(5,3)$ and $(5,-2)$ or state that the slope is undefined. Indicate if the line is horizontal or vertical.

Copyright © 2017 Pearson Education, Inc.

Learning Objective #2: Use slope to show that lines are parallel.

✔ Solved Problem #2

2. Show that the line passing through $(4, 2)$ and $(6, 6)$ is parallel to the line passing through $(0, -2)$ and $(1, 0)$.

Slope of line through (4,2) and (6,6):

$$m = \frac{\text{Change in } y}{\text{Change in } x} = \frac{6-2}{6-4} = \frac{4}{2} = 2$$

Slope of line through (0,–2) and (1,0):

$$m = \frac{\text{Change in } y}{\text{Change in } x} = \frac{0-(-2)}{1-0} = \frac{2}{1} = 2$$

Since their slopes are equal, the lines are parallel.

✎ Pencil Problem #2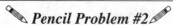

2. Determine if the line passing through $(-2, 0)$ and $(0, 6)$ is parallel to the line passing through $(1, 8)$ and $(0, 5)$.

Learning Objective #3: Use slope to show that lines are perpendicular.

✔ Solved Problem #3

3. Show that the line passing through $(-1, 4)$ and $(3, 2)$ is perpendicular to the line passing through $(-2, -1)$ and $(2, 7)$.

Line through (–1,4) and (3,2):

$$m = \frac{\text{Change in } y}{\text{Change in } x} = \frac{2-4}{3-(-1)}$$
$$= \frac{-2}{4}$$
$$= -\frac{1}{2}$$

Line through (–2,–1) and (2,7):

$$m = \frac{\text{Change in } y}{\text{Change in } x} = \frac{7-(-1)}{2-(-2)}$$
$$= \frac{8}{4}$$
$$= 2$$

Since the product of their slopes is $-\frac{1}{2}(2) = -1,$

the lines are perpendicular.

✎ Pencil Problem #3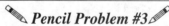

3. Determine if the line passing through $(1, 5)$ and $(0, 3)$ is perpendicular to the line passing through $(-2, 8)$ and $(2, 6)$.

Copyright © 2017 Pearson Education, Inc.

Learning Objective #4: Calculate rate of change in applied situations.

✔ *Solved Problem #4*	✏ *Pencil Problem #4* ✏

4. Use the ordered pairs in the figure shown to find the slope of the line segment that represents men. Express the slope correctly to two decimal places and describe what it represents.

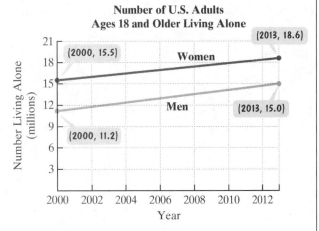

Number of U.S. Adults Ages 18 and Older Living Alone

4. Construction laws are very specific when it comes to access ramps for the disabled. The grade of a ramp refers to its slope expressed as a percent. Every vertical rise of 1 foot requires a horizontal run of 12 feet.

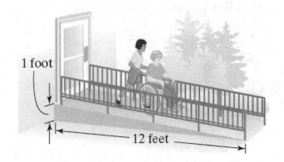

What is the grade of such a ramp? Round to the nearest tenth of a percent.

Let $(x_1, y_1) = (2000, 11.2)$ and $(x_2, y_2) = (2013, 15.0)$.

$$m = \frac{\text{Change in } y}{\text{Change in } x} = \frac{y_2 - y_1}{x_2 - x_1} = \frac{15.0 - 11.2}{2013 - 2000} = \frac{3.8}{13} \approx 0.29$$

The number of men living alone increased at a rate of 0.29 million per year.

The rate of change is 0.29 million men per year.

Answers for Pencil Problems *(Textbook Exercise references in parentheses)*:

1a. $m = \frac{3}{4}$ *(3.3 #1)* **1b.** $m = 0$; the line is horizontal *(3.3 #5)*

1c. the slope is undefined; the line is vertical *(3.3 #9)* **2.** parallel *(3.3 #23)*

3. perpendicular *(3.3 #27)* **4.** 8.3% *(3.3 #49)*

Homework:

☐ **Review the Section 3.3 summary** on page 273 of the textbook.

☐ **Insert your homework** into this section of the *Learning Guide*. Show all work neatly and check your answers. Strive to work through difficulties when possible, making note of any exercises where you need additional help. Remember, even if your instructor assigns homework through *MyMathLab*, you should still write out your work.

Copyright © 2017 Pearson Education, Inc.

Section 3.4
The Slope-Intercept Form of the Equation of a Line

FIRE and ICE!

Water freezes at 0° Celsius or at 32° Fahrenheit.
Water boils at 100° Celsius or at 212° Fahrenheit.

In this section, you will learn how to use this information to write a linear equation to express the relationship between Celsius temperature and Fahrenheit temperature.

First Steps:

☐ **Take comprehensive notes** from your instructor's lecture and insert your notes into this section of the *Learning Guide*. Be sure to write down all examples, definitions, and other key concepts. Additional learning resources include the *Video Lecture Series*, the *PowerPoints*, and Section 3.4 of your textbook which begins on page 245.

☐ Complete the **Concept and Vocabulary Check** on page 251 of the textbook.

Guided Practice:

☐ Review each of the following **Solved Problems** and complete each **Pencil Problem**.

Learning Objective #1: Find a line's slope and y-intercept from its equation.	
✔ **Solved Problem #1**	✎ **Pencil Problem #1** ✎
1a. Find the slope and the y-intercept of the line: $y = \dfrac{2}{3}x + 4$	**1a.** Find the slope and the y-intercept of the line: $y = -\dfrac{1}{2}x + 5$
The slope is the x-coefficient, which is $m = \dfrac{2}{3}$. The y-intercept is the constant term, which is 4.	
1b. Find the slope and the y-intercept of the line: $7x + y = 6$	**1b.** Find the slope and the y-intercept of the line: $3x + 2y = 3$
First, solve the equation for y. $7x + y = 6 \rightarrow y = -7x + 6$ The slope is the x-coefficient, which is $m = -7$. The y-intercept is the constant term, which is 6.	

Copyright © 2017 Pearson Education, Inc.

Learning Objective #2: Graph lines in slope-intercept form.

✔ *Solved Problem #2*

2a. Graph: $y = 3x - 2$

The y-intercept is –2, so plot the point $(0, -2)$.

The slope is $m = 3$ or $m = \dfrac{3}{1}$.

Find another point by going up 3 units and to the right 1 unit.

Use a straightedge to draw a line through the two points.

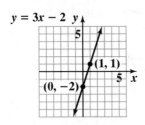

✎ *Pencil Problem #2* ✎

2a. Graph: $y = 2x + 4$

2b. Graph: $y = \dfrac{3}{5}x + 1$

The y-intercept is 1, so plot the point $(0,1)$.

The slope is $m = \dfrac{3}{5}$.

Find another point by going up 3 units and to the right 5 units.

Use a straightedge to draw a line through the two points.

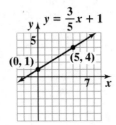

2b. Graph: $y = -\dfrac{3}{4}x + 2$

Copyright © 2017 Pearson Education, Inc.

Learning Objective #3: Use slope and y-intercept to graph $Ax + By = C$.

✔ Solved Problem #3

3. Graph $3x + 4y = 0$ by using slope and y-intercept.

Solve for y: $\quad 3x + 4y = 0$

$$4y = -3x$$

$$y = -\frac{3}{4}x$$

The y-intercept is 0, so plot the point $(0,0)$.

The slope is $m = \dfrac{-3}{4}$.

Find another point by going down 3 units and to the right 4 units.

Use a straightedge to draw a line through the two points.

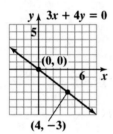

✎ Pencil Problem #3 ✎

3. Graph $7x + 2y = 14$ by using slope and y-intercept.

Learning Objective #4: Use slope and y-intercept to model data.

✔ Solved Problem #4

4. The figure shows the percentage of Americans who helped others or went shopping to improve their mood in 2003 and 2013..

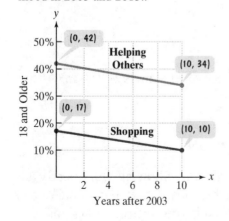

✎ Pencil Problem #4 ✎

4. The figure shows the racial and ethnic composition of the United States population in 2010, with projections for 2050.

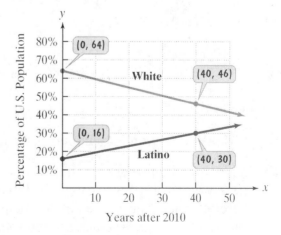

Copyright © 2017 Pearson Education, Inc.

4a. Use the two points for shopping in the figure to find an equation in the form $y = mx + b$ that models the percentage of Americans who improved their mood by shopping, y, x years after 2003.

The y-intercept is 17 and the slope is

$$m = \frac{\text{Change in } y}{\text{Change in } x} = \frac{10-17}{10-0} = \frac{-7}{10} = -0.7$$

The equation is $y = -0.7x + 17$.

4a. Use the two points for whites to find an equation in the form $y = mx + b$ that models the percentage of whites, y, in the United States population x years after 2010.
Round m to two decimal places.

4b. Use the model from part (a) to project the percentage of Americans who will improve their mood by shopping in 2023.

$$y = -0.7x + 17 = -0.7(20) + 17 = 3$$

The model projects that 3% of Americans will improve their mood by shopping in 2023.

4b. Use the model from part (a) to project the percentage of whites in the United States in 2110.

Answers for Pencil Problems *(Textbook Exercise references in parentheses)*:

1a. $m = -\dfrac{1}{2}$ and the y-intercept is 5 *(3.4 #5)* **1b.** $m = -\dfrac{3}{2}$ and the y-intercept is $\dfrac{3}{2}$ *(3.4 #23)*

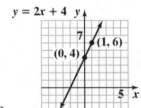

$y = 2x + 4$

2a. *(3.4 #27)*

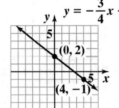

$y = -\dfrac{3}{4}x + 2$

2b. *(3.4 #35)*

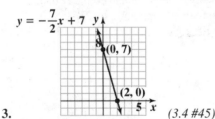

$y = -\dfrac{7}{2}x + 7$

3. *(3.4 #45)* **4a.** $y = -0.45x + 64$. *(3.4 #65a)* **4b.** 19% *(3.4 #65b)*

Homework:

☐ **Review the Section 3.4 summary** on page 274 of the textbook.

☐ **Insert your homework** into this section of the *Learning Guide*. Show all work neatly and check your answers. Strive to work through difficulties when possible, making note of any exercises where you need additional help. Remember, even if your instructor assigns homework through *MyMathLab*, you should still write out your work.

 Copyright © 2017 Pearson Education, Inc.

Section 3.5
The Point-Slope Form of the Equation of a Line

Cigarettes and Lung Cancer

Most people are surprised by the number of people that they see smoking cigarettes in movies and television shows made in the 1940s and 1950s. At that time, there was little awareness of the relationship between tobacco use and numerous diseases. Cigarette smoking was seen as a healthy way to relax and help digest a hearty meal.

Then, in 1964, a linear equation changed everything.

This scatter plot shows a relationship between cigarette consumption among males and deaths due to lung cancer per million males. The data are from 11 countries and date back to a 1964 report by the U.S. Surgeon General.

The scatter plot can be modeled by a line whose slope indicates an increasing death rate from lung cancer with increased cigarette consumption. At that time, the tobacco industry argued that in spite of this regression line, tobacco use is not the cause of cancer. Recent data do, indeed, show a causal effect between tobacco use and numerous diseases.

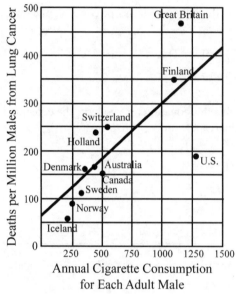

Source: Smoking and Health, Washington, D.C., 1964

The concepts that you learn in this section of your textbook will help you understand the mathematics behind this turning point in public health.

First Steps:

☐ **Take comprehensive notes** from your instructor's lecture and insert your notes into this section of the *Learning Guide*. Be sure to write down all examples, definitions, and other key concepts. Additional learning resources include the *Video Lecture Series*, the *PowerPoints*, and Section 3.5 of your textbook which begins on page 255.

☐ Complete the *Concept and Vocabulary Check* on page 260 of the textbook.

Copyright © 2017 Pearson Education, Inc.

Guided Practice:

☐ Review each of the following *Solved Problems* and complete each *Pencil Problem*.

Learning Objective #1: Use the point-slope form to write equations of a line.

✔ **Solved Problem #1**	✎ **Pencil Problem #1**
1a. Write the point-slope form and the slope-intercept form of the equation of the line with slope 6 that passes through the point $(2,-5)$.	**1a.** Write the point-slope form and the slope-intercept form of the equation of the line with slope -8 that passes through the point $(-3,-2)$.

1a. Begin by finding the point-slope equation of a line.

$$y - y_1 = m(x - x_1)$$
$$y - (-5) = 6(x - 2)$$
$$y + 5 = 6(x - 2)$$

Now solve this equation for y to write the equation in slope-intercept form.

$$y + 5 = 6(x - 2)$$
$$y + 5 = 6x - 12$$
$$y = 6x - 17$$

1b. A line passes through the points $(-2,-1)$ and $(-1,-6)$.

Find the equation of the line in point-slope form and in slope intercept form.

Begin by finding the slope: $m = \dfrac{-6-(-1)}{-1-(-2)} = \dfrac{-5}{1} = -5$

Using the slope and either point, find the point-slope equation of a line.

$$y - y_1 = m(x - x_1) \qquad \text{or} \qquad y - y_1 = m(x - x_1)$$
$$y - (-1) = -5(x - (-2)) \qquad \qquad y - (-6) = -5(x - (-1))$$
$$y + 1 = -5(x + 2) \qquad \qquad y + 6 = -5(x + 1)$$

To obtain slope-intercept form, solve the above equation for y:

$$y + 1 = -5(x + 2) \quad \text{or} \quad y + 6 = -5(x + 1)$$
$$y + 1 = -5x - 10 \qquad \qquad y + 6 = -5x - 5$$
$$y = -5x - 11 \qquad \qquad y = -5x - 11$$

1b. A line passes through the points $(-3,-1)$ and $(2,4)$.

Find the equation of the line in point-slope form and in slope-intercept form.

Copyright © 2017 Pearson Education, Inc.

Learning Objective #2: Write linear equations that model data and make predictions.

✔ Solved Problem #2

2. The bar graph below gives the median age of the U.S. population in the indicated year.

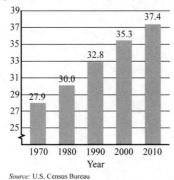

Source: U.S. Census Bureau

Here, the data are displayed as a set of five points in a rectangular coordinate system.

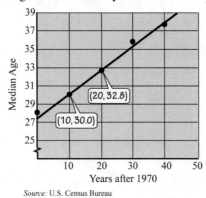

Source: U.S. Census Bureau

2a. Use the data points (10, 30.0) and (20, 32.8) from the figure to write the slope-intercept form of an equation that models the median age of the U.S. population x years after 1970.

First, find the slope: $m = \dfrac{32.8 - 30.0}{20 - 10} = \dfrac{2.8}{10} = 0.28$

Next, use the point-slope form to write the equation.

$y - y_1 = m(x - x_1)$

$y - 30.0 = 0.28(x - 10)$

Then solve for y to obtain slope-intercept form.

$y - 30.0 = 0.28(x - 10)$

$y - 30.0 = 0.28x - 2.8$

$\qquad y = 0.28x + 27.2$

✎ Pencil Problem #2 ✏

2. The bar graph shows the mean, or average, student loan debt in the United States, in 2011 dollars, for four selected years from 2001 through 2010.

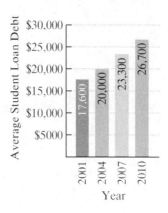

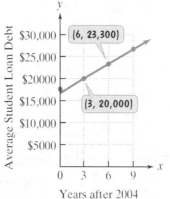

Source: Pew Research Center

2a. Shown below the bar graph is a scatter plot with a line passing through two of the data points. Use the two points whose coordinates are shown by the voice balloons to write the slope-intercept form of an equation that models the average student loan debt, y, in the United States x years after 2001.

2b. Use this model from part (a) to predict the median age in 2020.

2b. If trends shown by the data continue, use the model from part (a) to project the average student loan debt in 2021.

Because 2020 is 50 years after 1970, substitute 50 for x and compute y.

$$y = 0.28x + 27.2$$
$$= 0.28(50) + 27.2$$
$$= 14 + 27.2$$
$$= 41.2$$

The model predicts that 41.2 will be the median age in 2020.

Answers for Pencil Problems *(Textbook Exercise references in parentheses)*:

1a. point-slope form: $y + 2 = -8(x + 3)$; slope-intercept form: $y = -8x - 26$ *(3.5 #5)*

1b. point-slope form: $y + 1 = 1(x + 3)$ or $y - 4 = 1(x - 2)$; slope-intercept form: $y = x + 2$ *(3.5 #19)*

2a. $y = 1100x + 16,700$ *(3.5 #39a)*

2b. $38,700   *(3.5 #39b)*

Homework:

☐ **Review the Section 3.5 summary** on page 274 of the textbook.

☐ **Insert your homework** into this section of the *Learning Guide*. Show all work neatly and check your answers. Strive to work through difficulties when possible, making note of any exercises where you need additional help. Remember, even if your instructor assigns homework through *MyMathLab*, you should still write out your work.

Copyright © 2017 Pearson Education, Inc.

Section 3.6
Linear Inequalities in Two Variables

How much cholesterol?

An egg provides 165 milligrams of cholesterol and an ounce of meat provides 110 milligrams of cholesterol.

In this section of the textbook, we will explore an application of a linear inequality in two variables to help us to keep a patient from exceeding her daily cholesterol limit.

First Steps:

☐ **Take comprehensive notes** from your instructor's lecture and insert your notes into this section of the *Learning Guide*. Be sure to write down all examples, definitions, and other key concepts. Additional learning resources include the *Video Lecture Series*, the *PowerPoints*, and Section 3.6 of your textbook which begins on page 263.

☐ Complete the *Concept and Vocabulary Check* on page 269 of the textbook.

Guided Practice:

☐ Review each of the following *Solved Problems* and complete each *Pencil Problem*.

Learning Objective #1: Determine whether an ordered pair is a solution of an inequality.	
✔ *Solved Problem #1*	✎ *Pencil Problem #1* ✎
1a. Determine whether the ordered pair $(0,0)$ is a solution of the inequality $5x + 4y \le 20$.	**1a.** Determine whether the ordered pair $(0,0)$ is a solution of the inequality $2x + y \ge 5$.
Substitute 0 for x and 0 for y into the inequality. $$5x + 4y \le 20$$ $$5(0) + 4(0) \le 20$$ $$0 \le 20, \text{ true}$$ $(0,0)$ is a solution.	
1b. Determine whether the ordered pair $(6,2)$ is a solution of the inequality $5x + 4y \le 20$.	**1b.** Determine whether the ordered pair $(-2,-4)$ is a solution of the inequality $y \ge -2x + 4$.
Substitute 6 for x and 2 for y into the inequality. $$5x + 4y \le 20$$ $$5(6) + 4(2) \le 20$$ $$30 + 8 \le 20$$ $$38 \le 20, \text{ false}$$ $(6,2)$ is not a solution.	

Learning Objective #2: Graph a linear inequality in two variables.

✔ *Solved Problem #2*

2a. Graph: $2x - 4y < 8$

Step 1. Replace < with = and graph the linear equation $2x - 4y = 8$. Draw a dashed line because the inequality contains a < symbol.

Step 2. Use (0,0) as a test point.

$$2x - 4y < 8$$
$$2(0) - 4(0) < 8$$
$$0 < 8, \text{ true}$$

Step 3. The test point (0,0) is part of the solution set, so shade the half-plane containing (0,0).

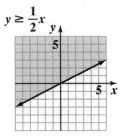

$2x - 4y < 8$

2b. Graph: $y \geq \dfrac{1}{2}x$

Step 1. Replace $\geq$ with = and graph the linear equation $y = \dfrac{1}{2}x$. The line passes through the origin so we must find an additional point. For example, using the slope we get the point (2,1). Draw a solid line because the inequality contains a $\geq$ symbol.

Step 2. We cannot use (0,0) as a test point because the line passes through it.

Use (0,10) as a test point $\quad y \geq \dfrac{1}{2}x$

$$10 \geq \dfrac{1}{2}(0)$$
$$10 \geq 0, \text{ true}$$

Step 3. The test point (0,10) is part of the solution set, so shade the half-plane containing (0,10).

$y \geq \dfrac{1}{2}x$

✎ *Pencil Problem #2*

2a. Graph: $x + 2y > 4$

2b. Graph: $y \leq \dfrac{1}{3}x$

Copyright © 2017 Pearson Education, Inc.

2c. Graph the inequality in a rectangular coordinate system: $y > 1$

Graph the horizontal line, $y = 1$, with a dashed line and shade the half-plane above the line.

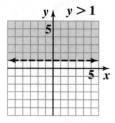

2c. Graph the inequality in a rectangular coordinate system: $y \leq -1$

2d. Graph the inequality in a rectangular coordinate system: $x \leq -2$

Graph the vertical line, $x = -2$, with a solid line and shade the half-plane to the left of the line.

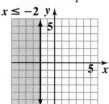

2d. Graph the inequality in a rectangular coordinate system: $x \geq 0$

Learning Objective #3: Solve applied problems involving linear inequalities in two variables.

✔ Solved Problem #3

3. Temperature and precipitation affect whether or not trees and forests can grow. At certain levels of precipitation and temperature, only grasslands and deserts will exist. The figure shows three kinds of regions—deserts, grasslands, and forests—that result from various ranges of temperature and precipitation. Notice that the horizontal axis is labeled T, for temperature, rather than x. The vertical axis is labeled P, for precipitation, rather than y.

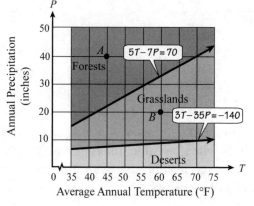

✏ Pencil Problem #3 ✏

3. Bottled water and medical supplies are to be shipped to survivors of a hurricane by plane. Each plane can carry no more than 80,000 pounds. The bottled water weighs 20 pounds per container and each medical kit weighs 10 pounds.

Let x represent the number of bottles of water to be shipped. Let y represent the number of medical kits.

The plane's weight limitations can be described by the following inequality:

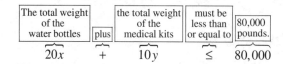

The total weight of the water bottles	plus	the total weight of the medical kits	must be less than or equal to	80,000 pounds.
$20x$	$+$	$10y$	$\leq$	$80,000$

Graph the inequality. Because x and y must be nonnegative, limit the graph to quadrant I and its boundary only.

Copyright © 2017 Pearson Education, Inc.

We can use inequalities in two variables, T and P, to describe the regions in the figure.

For average annual temperatures that exceed 35°F, the inequalities $5T - 7P \geq 70$ and $3T - 35P \leq -140$ model where grasslands occur. Show that the coordinates of point B satisfy both of these inequalities.

Substitute the coordinates of $B, (60, 20),$ into each inequality.

$$5T - 7P \geq 70$$
$$5(60) - 7(20) \geq 70$$
$$300 - 140 \geq 70$$
$$160 \geq 70, \ \text{true}$$

$$3T - 35P \leq -140$$
$$3(60) - 35(20) \leq -140$$
$$180 - 700 \leq -140$$
$$-520 \leq -140, \ \text{true}$$

Graph $20x + 10y \leq 80,000$

Answers for Pencil Problems *(Textbook Exercise references in parentheses)*:

1a. not a solution *(3.6 #3)*   **1b.** not a solution *(3.6 #5)*

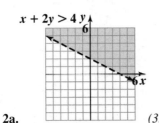

2a.   *(3.6 #13)*

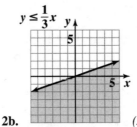

2b.   *(3.6 #23)*

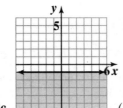

2c.   *(3.6 #43)*

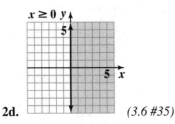

2d.   *(3.6 #35)*

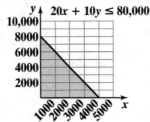

3.   *(3.6 #45)*

Homework:

☐ **Review the Section 3.6 summary** on page 275 of the textbook.

☐ **Insert your homework** into this section of the *Learning Guide*. Show all work neatly and check your answers. Strive to work through difficulties when possible, making note of any exercises where you need additional help. Remember, even if your instructor assigns homework through *MyMathLab*, you should still write out your work.

        Copyright © 2017 Pearson Education, Inc.

Group Project for Chapter 3

In Example 3 on page on page 259 of the textbook, we used the data in Figure 3.36 to develop a linear equation that modeled the graying of America. For this group exercise, you might find it helpful to pattern your work after Figure 3.36 and the solution to Example 3.

Group members should begin by consulting an almanac, newspaper, magazine, or the Internet to find data that lie approximately on or near a straight line. Working by hand or using a graphing utility, construct a scatter plot for the data. If working by hand, draw a line that passes through or near the data points and then write its equation. If using a graphing utility, obtain the equation of the regression line. Then use the equation of the line to make a prediction about what might happen in the future. Are there circumstances that might affect the accuracy of this prediction? List some of these circumstances.

Copyright © 2017 Pearson Education, Inc.

Getting Ready for the Chapter 3 Test

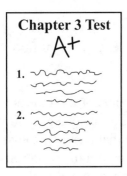

One of the best ways to prepare for a test is to stay on top of your studying, keeping up as your professor proceeds from section to section. Falling behind on one section often makes it difficult to understand the material in the following section. Never wait until the last minute to study for an exam.

Below are several actions that will help you stay organized as you prepare for your test.

How to prepare for your Chapter Test:

☐ **Write down any details that your instructor shares about the test.**
In addition to items such as location, date, time, and essentials to bring, be sure to listen carefully for specific information about the topics covered. Communicate with your instructor concerning any details that may be unclear to you.

☐ **Read the Chapter Summary that begins on page 272 of your textbook.**
Study the appropriate sections in the Chapter Summary. This summary contains the most important material in each section including, definitions, concepts, procedures, and examples.

☐ **Review your *Learning Guide*.**
Go back through the *Solved Problems* and *Pencil Problems* in this chapter of your *Learning Guide*. You may find it helpful to cover up solutions and work through the problems again.

☐ **Study your notes and homework.**
Read through your class notes that you took during this unit, and review the corresponding homework assignments.

☐ **Review quizzes and other feedback from your professor.**
Review any quizzes you have taken and be sure you understand any errors that you made. Seek help with any concepts that are still unclear.

☐ **Complete the Review Exercises that begin on page 275 of your textbook.**
Work the assigned problems from the Review Exercises. These exercises represent the most significant problems for each of the chapter's sections. The answers for all Review Exercises are in the back of your textbook.

☐ **Take the Chapter Test on page 278 of your textbook.**
- Find a quiet place to take the Chapter Test.
- Do not use notes, index cards, or any resources other than those your instructor will allow during the actual test.
- After completing the entire test, check your answers in the back of the textbook.
- Watch the *Chapter Test Prep Video* to review any exercises you may have missed.

          Copyright © 2017 Pearson Education, Inc.

Chapter 4.R Systems of Linear Equations and Inequalities
Integrated Review

Learning Objectives
1. Determine whether an ordered pair is a solution of an equation.

Learning Objective #1: Determine whether an ordered pair is a solution of an equation.

✔ **Solved Problem #1**	✎ **Pencil Problem #1** ✎
1a. Determine whether the ordered pair $(3, -2)$ is a solution of the equation $x - 3y = 9$.	**1a.** Determine whether the ordered pair $(0, 6)$ is a solution of the equation $y = 2x + 6$.

$$x - 3y = 9$$
$$3 - 3(-2) = 9$$
$$3 + 6 = 9$$
$$9 = 9, \text{ true}$$

$(3, -2)$ is a solution.

1b. Determine whether the ordered pair $(-2, 3)$ is a solution of the equation $x - 3y = 9$.

$$x - 3y = 9$$
$$-2 - 3(3) = 9$$
$$-2 - 9 = 9$$
$$-11 = 9, \text{ false}$$

$(-2, 3)$ is not a solution.

1b. Determine whether the ordered pair $(2, -2)$ is a solution of the equation $y = 2x + 6$.

Answers for Pencil Problems:

1a. $(0, 6)$ is a solution   **1b.** $(2, -2)$ is not a solution

Section 4.1
Solving Systems of Linear Equations by Graphing

The CO$T to Cross

Visitors to the world's great bridges are frequently inspired by their beauty.

This feeling is not always shared by daily commuters dealing with escalating toll costs and peak-hour congestion. For these frequent users, most bridge authorities provide the option of a fixed cost that reduces the toll. In this section, you will see how toll options in these situations can be modeled by two linear equations in two variables and their graphs.

First Steps:

☐ **Take comprehensive notes** from your instructor's lecture and insert your notes into this section of the *Learning Guide*. Be sure to write down all examples, definitions, and other key concepts. Additional learning resources include the *Video Lecture Series*, the *PowerPoints*, and Section 4.1 of your textbook which begins on page 282.

☐ Complete the *Concept and Vocabulary Check* on page 291 of the textbook.

Guided Practice:

☐ Review each of the following *Solved Problems* and complete each *Pencil Problem*.

Learning Objective #1: Decide whether an ordered pair is a solution of a linear system.

✔ Solved Problem #1

1. Determine if the ordered pair $(7,6)$ is a solution of the system: $\begin{cases} 2x - 3y = -4 \\ 2x + y = 4 \end{cases}$

To determine if $(7,6)$ is a solution to the system, replace x with 7 and y with 6 in both equations.

$$2x - 3y = -4 \qquad\qquad 2x + y = 4$$
$$2(7) - 3(6) = -4 \qquad\quad 2(7) + 6 = 4$$
$$14 - 18 = -4 \qquad\qquad 14 + 6 = 4$$
$$-4 = -4, \text{ true} \qquad\quad 20 = 4, \text{ false}$$

The ordered pair does not satisfy both equations, so it is not a solution to the system.

✎ Pencil Problem #1 ✎

1. Determine if the ordered pair $(2,-3)$ is a solution of the system: $\begin{cases} 2x + 3y = -5 \\ 7x - 3y = 23 \end{cases}$

Copyright © 2017 Pearson Education, Inc.

Learning Objective #2: Solve systems of linear equations by graphing.

✔ **Solved Problem #2**   ✎ **Pencil Problem #2**✎

2. Solve by graphing: $\begin{cases} 2x + y = 6 \\ 2x - y = -2 \end{cases}$

2. Solve by graphing: $\begin{cases} x + y = 1 \\ y - x = 3 \end{cases}$

Graph $2x + y = 6$ by using intercepts.

x-intercept (Set $y = 0$.)

$2x + y = 6$

$2x + 0 = 6$

$2x = 6$

$x = 3$

y-intercept (Set $x = 0$.)

$2x + y = 6$

$2(0) + y = 6$

$0 + y = 6$

$y = 6$

Graph $2x - y = -2$ by using intercepts.

x-intercept (Set $y = 0$.)

$2x - y = -2$

$2x - 0 = -2$

$2x = -2$

$x = -1$

y-intercept (Set $x = 0$.)

$2x - y = -2$

$2(0) - y = -2$

$-y = -2$

$y = 2$

Graph both lines:

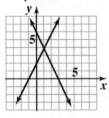

The lines intersect at (1,4).

The solution set is $\{(1,4)\}$.

Copyright © 2017 Pearson Education, Inc.

Learning Objective #3:
Use graphing to identify systems with no solution or infinitely many solutions.

✔ Solved Problem #3

3a. Solve by graphing: $\begin{cases} y = 3x - 2 \\ y = 3x + 1 \end{cases}$

Graph $y = 3x - 2$ by using the y-intercept of –2 and the slope of 3.

Graph $y = 3x + 1$ by using the y-intercept of 1 and the slope of 3.

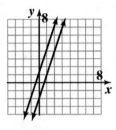

Because both equations have the same slope, 3, but different y-intercepts, the lines are parallel.

Thus, the system is inconsistent and has no solution.

The solution set is the empty set, $\{\ \}$.

✎ Pencil Problem #3✎

3a. Solve by graphing: $\begin{cases} y = 2x - 1 \\ y = 2x + 1 \end{cases}$

3b. Solve by graphing: $\begin{cases} x + y = 3 \\ 2x + 2y = 6 \end{cases}$

Graph $x + y = 3$ by using intercepts.

x-intercept (Set $y = 0.$) y-intercept (Set $x = 0.$)
$x + y = 3$ $x + y = 3$
$x + 0 = 3$ $0 + y = 3$
$\quad x = 3$ $\quad y = 3$

Graph $2x + 2y = 6$ by using intercepts.

x-intercept (Set $y = 0.$) y-intercept (Set $x = 0.$)
$2x + 2y = 6$ $2x + 2y = 6$
$2x + 2(0) = 6$ $2(0) + 2y = 6$
$\quad 2x = 6$ $\quad 2y = 6$
$\quad\ x = 3$ $\quad\ y = 3$

Both lines have the same x-intercept and the same y-intercept.

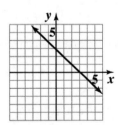

Thus, the graphs of the two equations in the system are the same line.

Any ordered pair that is a solution to one equation is a solution to the other, and, consequently, a solution of the system. The system has an infinite number of solutions, namely all points that are solutions of either line.

The solution set is $\{(x, y) \mid x + y = 3\}$.

3b. Solve by graphing: $\begin{cases} x - 2y = 4 \\ 2x - 4y = 8 \end{cases}$

Copyright © 2017 Pearson Education, Inc.

Learning Objective #4: Use graphs of linear systems to solve problems.

✔ *Solved Problem #4* | ✎ *Pencil Problem #4*✎

4. The toll to a bridge costs $2.00. If you use the bridge x times in a month, the monthly cost, y, is $y = 2x$.

With a $10 discount pass, the toll is reduced to $1.00. The monthly cost, y, of using the bridge x times in a month with the discount pass is $y = x + 10$.

4. You plan to start taking an aerobics class. Nonmembers pay $4 per class. Members pay a $10 monthly fee plus an additional $2 per class. The monthly cost, y, of taking x classes can be modeled by the linear system $\begin{cases} y = 4x \\ y = 2x + 10 \end{cases}$

4a. Solve by graphing the system: $\begin{cases} y = 2x \\ y = x + 10 \end{cases}$

Suggestion: Let the x-axis extend from 0 to 20 and let the y-axis extend from 0 to 40.

4a. Solve the system by graphing.

Graph $y = 2x$ by using the y-intercept of 0 and the slope of 2.

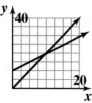

Graph $y = x + 10$ by using the y-intercept of 10 and the slope of 1.

The solution is the ordered pair (10,20).

4b. Interpret the coordinates of the solution in practical terms.

4b. Interpret the coordinates of the solution in practical terms.

If the bridge is used 10 times in a month, the total monthly cost without the discount pass is the same as the monthly cost with the discount pass, namely $20.

Answers for Pencil Problems *(Textbook Exercise references in parentheses)*:

1. $(2, -3)$ is a solution of the system   *(4.1 #1)*   **2.** $\{(-1, 2)\}$ *(4.1 #13)*   **3a.** no solution or $\{\ \}$ *(4.1 #25)*

3b. infinitely many solutions; $\{(x, y) | x - 2y = 4\}$ or $\{(x, y) | 2x - 4y = 8\}$.   *(4.1 #29)*   **4a.** $\{(5, 20)\}$ *(4.1 #53a)*

4b. Nonmembers and members pay the same amount per month for taking 5 classes, namely $20.   *(4.1 #53b)*

Homework:

☐ **Review the Section 4.1 summary** on page 335 of the textbook.

☐ **Insert your homework** into this section of the *Learning Guide*. Show all work neatly and check your answers. Strive to work through difficulties when possible, making note of any exercises where you need additional help. Remember, even if your instructor assigns homework through *MyMathLab*, you should still write out your work.

   Copyright © 2017 Pearson Education, Inc.

Section 4.2
Solving Systems of Linear Equations by the Substitution Method

Pay at the Pump !

What is going on at the gas pumps? Prices seem to be going up and down...but mostly up! Like all things in a free-market economy, the price of a commodity is based on supply and demand.

In this section, we use a second method for solving linear systems, the substitution method, to understand this economic phenomenon.

First Steps:

☐ **Take comprehensive notes** from your instructor's lecture and insert your notes into this section of the *Learning Guide*. Be sure to write down all examples, definitions, and other key concepts. Additional learning resources include the *Video Lecture Series*, the *PowerPoints*, and Section 4.2 of your textbook which begins on page 294.

☐ Complete the ***Concept and Vocabulary Check*** on page 300 of the textbook.

Guided Practice:

☐ Review each of the following *Solved Problems* and complete each *Pencil Problem*.

Learning Objective #1: Solve linear systems by the substitution method.	
✔ *Solved Problem #1*	✎ *Pencil Problem #1*✎

1a. Solve by the substitution method:

$$\begin{cases} y = 5x - 13 \\ 2x + 3y = 12 \end{cases}$$

Since the first equation is solved for y, substitute $5x - 13$ for y in the second equation.

$$2x + 3(\overbrace{5x - 13}^{y}) = 12$$
$$2x + 15x - 39 = 12$$
$$17x - 39 = 12$$
$$17x = 51$$
$$x = 3$$

Back-substitute 3 for x into the first equation.
$$y = 5x - 13$$
$$y = 5(3) - 13$$
$$= 2$$

The solution set is $\{(3, 2)\}$.

1a. Solve by the substitution method:

$$\begin{cases} x + 3y = 8 \\ y = 2x - 9 \end{cases}$$

1b. Solve by the substitution method:

$$\begin{cases} 3x + 2y = -1 \\ x - y = 3 \end{cases}$$

Solve the second equation for x.

$x - y = 3$

$\quad x = y + 3$

Substitute $y + 3$ for x in the first equation.

$\quad 3x + 2y = -1$

$3(\overbrace{y+3}^{x}) + 2y = -1$

$\quad 3y + 9 + 2y = -1$

$\quad\quad 5y + 9 = -1$

$\quad\quad\quad 5y = -10$

$\quad\quad\quad\quad y = -2$

Back-substitute -2 for y into $x = y + 3$.

$x = y + 3$

$x = -2 + 3 = 1$

The solution set is $\{(1, -2)\}$.

1b. Solve by the substitution method:

$$\begin{cases} 2x - y = -5 \\ x + 5y = 14 \end{cases}$$

Learning Objective #2:
Use the substitution method to identify systems with no solution or infinitely many solutions.

✔ **Solved Problem #2**

✎ **Pencil Problem #2**✎

2a. Solve by the substitution method:

$$\begin{cases} 3x + y = -5 \\ y = -3x + 3 \end{cases}$$

Since the second equation is solved for y, substitute $-3x + 3$ for y in the first equation.

$\quad 3x + y \quad = -5$

$3x + (\overbrace{-3x+3}^{y}) = -5$

$\quad 3x - 3x + 3 = -5$

$\quad\quad\quad 3 = -5, \ \text{false}$

The false statement indicates that the system is inconsistent and has no solution.

The solution set is $\{\ \}$.

2a. Solve by the substitution method:

$$\begin{cases} x = 9 - 2y \\ x + 2y = 13 \end{cases}$$

Copyright © 2017 Pearson Education, Inc.

2b. Solve by the substitution method:
$$\begin{cases} y = 3x - 4 \\ 9x - 3y = 12 \end{cases}$$

Substitute $3x - 4$ for y in the second equation.

$$9x - 3y = 12$$

$$9x - 3(\overbrace{3x - 4}^{y}) = 12$$
$$9x - 9x + 12 = 12$$
$$12 = 12, \text{ true}$$

The true statement indicates that the system contains dependent equations and has infinitely many solutions.

The solution set is $\{(x, y) \mid y = 3x - 4\}$ or $\{(x, y) \mid 9x - 3y = 12\}$.

2b. Solve by the substitution method:
$$\begin{cases} y = 3x - 5 \\ 21x - 35 = 7y \end{cases}$$

Learning Objective #3: Solve problems using the substitution method.

✔ *Solved Problem #3*

3. The following models describe demand and supply for two-bedroom rental apartments, where p is the monthly rental price and x is the number of apartments.

Demand Model	Supply Model
$p = -30x + 1800$	$p = 30x$

3a. Solve the system and find the equilibrium quantity and the equilibrium price.

Substitute $30x$ for p in the first equation.

$$p = -30x + 1800$$

$$\overbrace{30x}^{p} = -30x + 1800$$
$$60x = 1800$$
$$x = 30$$

Back-substitute to find p.
$$p = 30x$$
$$p = 30(30) = 900$$

The solution set is $\{(30, 900)\}$.

Equilibrium quantity: 30
Equilibrium price: $900

✎ *Pencil Problem #3* ✎

3. The following models describe the price of a gallon of gasoline, where p is the price per gallon and x is the number of gallons demanded per day.

Demand Model	Supply Model
$p = -0.002x + 6$	$p = 0.001x + 3$

3a. Solve the system and find the equilibrium quantity and the equilibrium price for a gallon of gasoline.

3b. Use your answer from part (a) to complete this statement:

When rents are _____ per month, consumers

will demand _____ apartments and suppliers will

offer _____ apartments for rent.

When rents are $900 per month, consumers will demand 30 apartments and suppliers will offer 30 apartments for rent.

3b. Use your answer from part (a) to complete the statement:

If gasoline is sold for _____ per gallon, there will

be a demand for _____ gallons per day and

_____ gallons will be supplied per day.

Answers for Pencil Problems *(Textbook Exercise references in parentheses)*:

1a. $\{(5,1)\}$ *(4.2 #3)*

1b. $\{(-1,3)\}$ *(4.2 #7)*

2a. no solution or $\{\ \}$ *(4.2 #13)*

2b. infinitely many solutions or $\{(x,y)\,|\,y=3x-5\}$ or $\{(x,y)\,|\,21x-35=7y\}$ *(4.2 #15)*

3a. Ordered pair: (1000,4). Equilibrium number of gallons: 1000 gallons Equilibrium per gallon: $4.00   *(4.2 #41a)*

3b. If unleaded premium gasoline is sold for $4 per gallon, there will be a demand for 1000 gallons per day and 1000 gallons will be supplied per day.   *(4.2 #41b)*

Homework:

☐ **Review the Section 4.2 summary** on page 336 of the textbook.

☐ **Insert your homework** into this section of the *Learning Guide*. Show all work neatly and check your answers. Strive to work through difficulties when possible, making note of any exercises where you need additional help. Remember, even if your instructor assigns homework through *MyMathLab*, you should still write out your work.

Copyright © 2017 Pearson Education, Inc.

Section 4.3
Solving Systems of Linear Equations by the Addition Method

Procrastination makes you sick!

Researchers compared college students who were procrastinators and nonprocrastinators. Early in the semester, procrastinators reported fewer symptoms of illness, but late in the semester, they reported more symptoms than their nonprocrastinating peers.

In this section of the textbook, a third solution method, called addition, will verify (6, 3.5) as the point of intersection.

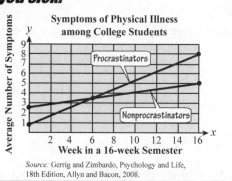

Source: Gerrig and Zimbardo, Psychology and Life, 18th Edition, Allyn and Bacon, 2008.

First Steps:

☐ **Take comprehensive notes** from your instructor's lecture and insert your notes into this section of the *Learning Guide*. Be sure to write down all examples, definitions, and other key concepts. Additional learning resources include the *Video Lecture Series*, the *PowerPoints*, and Section 4.3 of your textbook which begins on page 303.

☐ Complete the *Concept and Vocabulary Check* on page 309 of the textbook.

Guided Practice:

☐ Review each of the following *Solved Problems* and complete each *Pencil Problem*.

Learning Objective #1: Solve linear systems by the addition method.

✔ *Solved Problem #1*	✏ *Pencil Problem #1* ✏

1a. Solve the system: $\begin{cases} x + y = 5 \\ x - y = 9 \end{cases}$

Add the equations to eliminate the y-terms.

$x + y = 5$

$\underline{x - y = 9}$

$2x \quad = 14$

Now solve for x.

$2x = 14$

$x = 7$

Back-substitute into either of the original equations to solve for y.

$x + y = 5$

$7 + y = 5$

$y = -2$

The solution set is $\{(7, -2)\}$.

1a. Solve the system: $\begin{cases} x + y = -3 \\ x - y = 11 \end{cases}$

Copyright © 2017 Pearson Education, Inc.

1b. Solve the system: $\begin{cases} 4x - y = 22 \\ 3x + 4y = 26 \end{cases}$

Multiply each term of the first equation by 4 and add the equations to eliminate y.

$$16x - 4y = 88$$
$$\underline{3x + 4y = 26}$$
$$19x \qquad = 114$$
$$x = 6$$

Back-substitute into either of the original equations to solve for y.
$$4x - y = 22$$
$$4(6) - y = 22$$
$$24 - y = 22$$
$$-y = -2$$
$$y = 2$$

The solution set is $\{(6, 2)\}$.

1b. Solve the system: $\begin{cases} 3x + y = 7 \\ 2x - 5y = -1 \end{cases}$

1c. Solve the system: $\begin{cases} 4x + 5y = 3 \\ 2x - 3y = 7 \end{cases}$

Multiply each term of the second equation by –2 and add the equations to eliminate x.
$$4x + 5y = 3$$
$$\underline{-4x + 6y = -14}$$
$$11y = -11$$
$$y = -1$$

Back-substitute into either of the original equations to solve for x.
$$2x - 3y = 7$$
$$2x - 3(-1) = 7$$
$$2x + 3 = 7$$
$$2x = 4$$
$$x = 2$$

The solution set is $\{(2, -1)\}$.

1c. Solve the system: $\begin{cases} 3x - 4y = 11 \\ 2x + 3y = -4 \end{cases}$

Copyright © 2017 Pearson Education, Inc.

1d. Solve the system: $\begin{cases} 2x = 9 + 3y \\ 4y = 8 - 3x \end{cases}$

Rewrite each equation in the form $Ax + By = C$.

$2x - 3y = 9$

$3x + 4y = 8$

Multiply the top equation by 4 and multiply the bottom equation by 3.

$8x - 12y = 36$

$\underline{9x + 12y = 24}$

$17x \qquad = 60$

$\qquad x = \dfrac{60}{17}$

Back-substitution of $\dfrac{60}{17}$ to find y would cause cumbersome arithmetic. Instead, use the system that is in the form $Ax + By = C$ to eliminate x and find y.

$2x - 3y = 9$

$3x + 4y = 8$

Multiply the top equation by -3 and multiply the bottom equation by 2.

$-6x + 9y = -27$

$\underline{6x + 8y = \ 16}$

$\qquad 17y = -11$

$\qquad\quad y = \dfrac{-11}{17}$

The solution set is $\left\{ \left(\dfrac{60}{17}, -\dfrac{11}{17} \right) \right\}$.

1d. Solve the system: $\begin{cases} 2x - y = 3 \\ 4x + 4y = -1 \end{cases}$

Learning Objective #2:
Use the addition method to identify systems with no solution or infinitely many solutions.

✔ **Solved Problem #2**

2a. Solve the system: $\begin{cases} x + 2y = 4 \\ 3x + 6y = 13 \end{cases}$

Multiply the first equation by -3 and then add.

$-3x - 6y = -12$

$\underline{3x + 6y = \ 13}$

$\qquad 0 = \ \ 1, \text{ false}$

The false statement indicates that the system is inconsistent and has no solution.

The solution set is $\{\ \}$.

✎ **Pencil Problem #2** ✎

2a. Solve the system: $\begin{cases} 3x - y = 1 \\ 3x - y = 2 \end{cases}$

2b. Solve the system: $\begin{cases} x - 5y = 7 \\ 3x - 15y = 21 \end{cases}$

Multiply the first equation by −3 and then add.

$$-3x + 15y = -21$$
$$\underline{3x - 15y = 21}$$
$$0 = 0, \text{ true}$$

The true statement indicates that the system has infinitely many solutions.

The solution set is $\{(x, y) | x - 5y = 7\}$ or $\{(x, y) | 3x - 15y = 21\}$.

2b. Solve the system: $\begin{cases} x + 3y = 2 \\ 3x + 9y = 6 \end{cases}$

| **Learning Objective #3:** Determine the most efficient method for solving a linear system. |

✔ Solved Problem #3

3. True or False: If the solutions of a linear system do not involve integers, then it can be difficult to determine the exact solution when using the Graphing Method.

True

✏ Pencil Problem #3 ✏

3. True or False: The Substitution Method is often the best choice when solving a linear system that has an equation with a variable that is on one side by itself.

Answers for Pencil Problems *(Textbook Exercise references in parentheses)*:

1a. $\{(4, -7)\}$ *(4.3 #1)* **1b.** $\{(2, 1)\}$ *(4.3 #9)* **1c.** $\{(1, -2)\}$ *(4.3 #17)* **1d.** $\left\{\left(\dfrac{11}{12}, -\dfrac{7}{6}\right)\right\}$ *(4.3 #25)*

2a. no solution or { } *(4.3 #29)*

2b. The solution set is $\{(x, y) | x + 3y = 2\}$ or $\{(x, y) | 3x + 9y = 6\}$. *(4.3 #31)*

3. true *(4.3 #79)*

Homework:

☐ **Review the Section 4.3 summary** on page 336 of the textbook.

☐ **Insert your homework** into this section of the *Learning Guide*. Show all work neatly and check your answers. Strive to work through difficulties when possible, making note of any exercises where you need additional help. Remember, even if your instructor assigns homework through *MyMathLab*, you should still write out your work.

Copyright © 2017 Pearson Education, Inc.

Section 4.4
Problem Solving Using Systems of Equations

Talk! Talk! Talk!

Many Americans say they cannot live without their cell phones. Whether it is for talking, texting, or using data, we seem to be obsessed. But choosing the best plan can be difficult.

In this section of the textbook, we will explore the question of
"Which plan is most cost effective?" from a mathematical viewpoint.

First Steps:

☐ **Take comprehensive notes** from your instructor's lecture and insert your notes into this section of the *Learning Guide*. Be sure to write down all examples, definitions, and other key concepts. Additional learning resources include the *Video Lecture Series*, the *PowerPoints*, and Section 4.4 of your textbook which begins on page 313.

☐ Complete the *Concept and Vocabulary Check* on page 323 of the textbook.

Guided Practice:

☐ Review each of the following *Solved Problems* and complete each *Pencil Problem*.

Learning Objective #1: Solve problems using linear systems.

✔ *Solved Problem #1*

1a. Socializing is a favorite leisure activity. Each weekend day, the sum of the average times spent socializing for men and women is 138 minutes. The difference between the average times spent socializing for women and men is 8 minutes. How many minutes per day on weekends do men and women devote to socializing?

Let x = average time per day women spend socializing.
Let y = average time per day men spend socializing.

$$x + y = 138$$
$$\underline{x - y = 8}$$
$$2x = 146$$
$$x = 73$$

Back-substitute 73 for x to find y.
$$x + y = 138$$
$$73 + y = 138$$
$$y = 65$$

Men average 65 minutes per day socializing and women average 73 minutes.

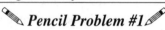 *Pencil Problem #1*

1a. Each day, the sum of the average times spent on grooming for 20- to 24-year-old women and men is 86 minutes. The difference between grooming times for 20- to 24-year-old women and men is 12 minutes. How many minutes per day do 20- to 24-year-old women and men spend on grooming?

Copyright © 2017 Pearson Education, Inc.

1b. A rectangular lot whose perimeter is 360 feet is fenced along three sides.

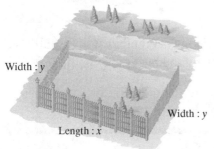

Width : y

Width : y

Length : x

An expensive fencing along the lot's length costs $20 per foot. An inexpensive fencing along the two side widths costs only $8 per foot. The total cost of the fencing along the three sides comes to $3280. What are the lot's dimensions?

Let x = the length of the lot.
Let y = the width of the lot.

Use the formula for the perimeter of a rectangle to write the first equation.
$$P = 2l + 2w$$
$$360 = 2x + 2y$$

Use the other information in the problem to write the second equation.
$$20x + 8 \cdot 2y = 3280$$

The two equations form the system.
$$\begin{cases} 2x + 2y = 360 \\ 20x + 16y = 3280 \end{cases}$$

Multiply the first equation by -8 and add the result to the second equation.
$$-16x - 16y = -2880$$
$$\underline{20x + 16y = 3280}$$
$$\begin{aligned} 4x &= 400 \\ x &= 100 \end{aligned}$$

Back-substitute to find y.
$$\begin{aligned} 2x + 2y &= 360 \\ 2(100) + 2y &= 360 \\ 200 + 2y &= 360 \\ 2y &= 160 \\ y &= 80 \end{aligned}$$

The length is 100 feet and the width is 80 feet.

1b. A rectangular lot whose perimeter is 320 feet is fenced along three sides. An expensive fencing along the lot's length costs $16 per foot. An inexpensive fencing along the two side widths costs only $5 per foot. The total cost of the fencing along the three sides comes to $2140. What are the lot's dimensions?

Copyright © 2017 Pearson Education, Inc.

Learning Objective #2: Solve simple interest problems.

| ✔ Solved Problem #2 | ✎ Pencil Problem #2 ✐ |

2. Suppose that you invested $25,000, part at 9% simple interest and the remainder at 12%. If the total yearly interest from these investments was $2550, find the amount invested at each rate.

Let x = the amount invested at 9%.
Let y = the amount invested at 12%.

$$\begin{cases} x + y = 25,000 \\ 0.09x + 0.12y = 2550 \end{cases}$$

This system can be solved by substitution.
Solve for y in terms of x.

$x + y = 25,000$

$\quad y = -x + 25,000$

Substitute this value into the other equation.

$$0.09x + 0.12y = 2550$$

$$0.09x + 0.12(\overbrace{-x + 25,000}^{y}) = 2550$$

$$0.09x - 0.12x + 3000 = 2550$$

$$-0.03x + 3000 = 2550$$

$$-0.03x = -450$$

$$x = 15,000$$

Back-substitute to find y.

$y = -x + 25,000$

$y = -(15,000) + 25,000$

$y = 10,000$

There was $15,000 invested at 9% and $10,000 invested at 12%.

2. A bank loaned out $120,000, part of it at the rate of 8% annual mortgage interest and the rest at the rate of 18% annual credit card interest. The interest received on both loans totaled $10,000. How much was loaned at each rate?

Learning Objective #3: Solve mixture problems.

✔ Solved Problem #3

3. A chemist needs to mix a 10% acid solution with a 60% acid solution to obtain 50 milliliters of a 30% acid solution. How many milliliters of each of the acid solutions must be used?

Let x = the number of milliliters of 10% acid solution.
Let y = the number of milliliters of 60% acid solution.

$$\begin{cases} x+y=50 \\ 0.10x+0.60y=0.30(50) \end{cases}$$

This system can be solved by substitution.
Solve for y in terms of x.
$x+y=50$

$\qquad y=-x+50$

Substitute this value into the other equation.
$$0.10x+0.60y=0.30(50)$$
$$0.10x+0.60y=15$$

$$0.10x+0.60(\overset{y}{\overbrace{-x+50}})=15$$
$$0.10x-0.60x+30=15$$
$$-0.50x+30=15$$
$$-0.50x=-15$$
$$x=30$$

Back-substitute to find y.
$y=-x+50$

$y=-(30)+50$

$y=20$

The chemist should mix 30 milliliters of the 10% acid solution and 20 milliliters of the 60% acid solution.

✎ Pencil Problem #3 ✎

3. A lab technician needs to mix a 5% fungicide solution with a 10% fungicide solution to obtain a 50-liter mixture consisting of 8% fungicide. How many liters of each of the fungicide solutions must be used?

Answers for Pencil Problems *(Textbook Exercise references in parentheses)*:

1a. 20- to 24-year-old women averaged 49 minutes grooming and men averaged 37 minutes. *(4.4 #5)*

1b. 90 feet by 70 feet *(4.4 #15)*   **2.** $116,000 was loaned at 8% and $4000 was loaned at 18%. *(4.4 #31)*

3. 20 liters of 5% fungicide solution and 30 liters of 10% fungicide solution *(4.4 #37)*

Homework:

☐ **Review the Section 4.4 summary** on page 336 of the textbook.

☐ **Insert your homework** into this section of the *Learning Guide*. Show all work neatly and check your answers. Strive to work through difficulties when possible, making note of any exercises where you need additional help. Remember, even if your instructor assigns homework through *MyMathLab*, you should still write out your work.

  Copyright © 2017 Pearson Education, Inc.

Section 4.5
Systems of Linear Inequalities

Does Your Weight Fit You?

This chapter opened by noting that the modern emphasis on thinness as the ideal body shape has been suggested as a major cause of eating disorders.

In this section, the textbook will demonstrate how systems of linear inequalities in two variables can enable you to establish a healthy weight range for your height and age.

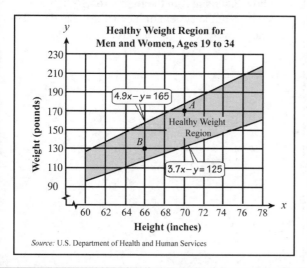

Healthy Weight Region for Men and Women, Ages 19 to 34

Source: U.S. Department of Health and Human Services

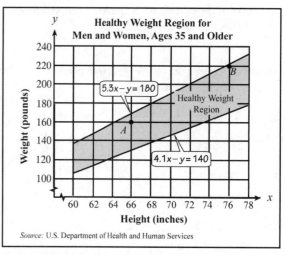

Healthy Weight Region for Men and Women, Ages 35 and Older

Source: U.S. Department of Health and Human Services

First Steps:

☐ **Take comprehensive notes** from your instructor's lecture and insert your notes into this section of the *Learning Guide*. Be sure to write down all examples, definitions, and other key concepts. Additional learning resources include the *Video Lecture Series*, the *PowerPoints*, and Section 4.5 of your textbook which begins on page 329.

☐ Complete the *Concept and Vocabulary Check* on page 332 of the textbook.

Guided Practice:

☐ Review each of the following *Solved Problems* and complete each *Pencil Problem*.

Copyright © 2017 Pearson Education, Inc.

Learning Objective #1: Use mathematical models involving systems of linear inequalities.

✔ *Solved Problem #1*

1. The healthy weight region for men and women ages 19 to 34 shown in the figure on the previous page can be modeled by the following system of linear inequalities:

$$\begin{cases} 4.9x - y \geq 165 \\ 3.7x - y \leq 125 \end{cases}$$

Show that point B in the figure, $(66,130)$, is a solution of the system of inequalities that describes healthy weight for this age group.

Substitute the coordinates of point B into both inequalities of the system.

$$\begin{cases} 4.9x - y \geq 165 \\ 3.7x - y \leq 125 \end{cases}$$

Point $B = (66,130)$

$$4.9x - y \geq 165$$
$$4.9(66) - 130 \geq 165$$
$$193.4 \geq 165, \text{ true}$$

$$3.7x - y \leq 125$$
$$3.7(66) - 130 \leq 125$$
$$114.2 \leq 125, \text{ true}$$

Point B is a solution of the system.

✎ *Pencil Problem #1*

1. The healthy weight region for men and women ages 35 and older shown in the figure on the previous page can be modeled by the following system of linear inequalities:

$$\begin{cases} 5.3x - y \geq 180 \\ 4.1x - y \leq 14 \end{cases}$$

Show that point A in the figure, $(66,160)$, is a solution of the system of inequalities that describes healthy weight for this age group.

Learning Objective #2: Graph the solution sets of systems of linear inequalities.

✔ *Solved Problem #2*

2a. Graph the solution set of the system:
$$\begin{cases} x + 2y > 4 \\ 2x - 3y \leq -6 \end{cases}$$

Graph $x + 2y > 4$ by graphing $x + 2y = 4$ as a dashed line using the x-intercept, 4, and the y-intercept, 2.

Use $(0,0)$ as a test point. $x + 2y > 4$
$$0 + 2(0) > 4$$
$$0 > 4, \text{ false}$$

Because $0 + 2(0) > 4$ is false, shade the half-plane *not* containing $(0,0)$.

✎ *Pencil Problem #2*

2a. Graph the solution set of the system:
$$\begin{cases} x - 2y > 4 \\ 2x + y \geq 6 \end{cases}$$

Copyright © 2017 Pearson Education, Inc.

Graph $2x - 3y \le -6$ by graphing $2x - 3y = -6$ as a solid line using the x-intercept, -3, and the y-intercept, 2.

Use $(0,0)$ as a test point.
$$2x - 3y \le -6$$
$$2(0) - 3(0) \le -6$$
$$0 \le -6, \text{ false}$$

Because $2(0) - 3(0) \le -6$ is false, shade the half-plane *not* containing $(0,0)$.

The solution set of the system is the intersection of the two shaded regions.

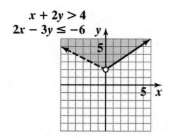

$$x + 2y > 4$$
$$2x - 3y \le -6$$

2b. Graph the solution set of the system:
$$\begin{cases} y \ge x + 2 \\ x \ge 1 \end{cases}$$

Graph $y \ge x + 2$ by graphing $y = x + 2$ as a solid line using the y-intercept, 2, and the slope, 1.

Use $(0,0)$ as a test point. $y \ge x + 2$
$$0 \ge 0 + 2$$
$$0 \ge 2, \text{ false}$$

Because $0 \ge 0 + 2$ is false, shade the half-plane *not* containing $(0,0)$.

Graph $x \ge 1$ by graphing $x = 1$ as a solid vertical line through $x = 1$.

Use $(0,0)$ as a test point. $x \ge 1$
$$0 \ge 1, \text{ false}$$

2b. Graph the solution set of the system:
$$\begin{cases} x + y > 1 \\ x + y < 4 \end{cases}$$

Because $0 \geq 1$ is false, shade the half-plane *not* containing $(0,0)$.

The solution set of the system is the intersection of the two shaded regions.

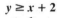
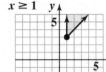

Answers for Pencil Problems *(Textbook Exercise references in parentheses)*:

1. $5.3x - y \geq 180$ $4.1x - y \leq 14$ *(4.5 #45)*

 $5.3(66) - 160 \geq 180$ $4.1(66) - 160 \leq 140$

  $189.8 \geq 180,$ true $110.6 \leq 140,$ true

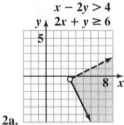

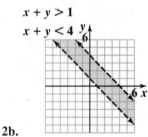

2a.   *(4.5 #7)*   **2b.**   *(4.5 #9)*

Homework:

☐ **Review the Section 4.5 summary** on page 337 of the textbook.

☐ **Insert your homework** into this section of the *Learning Guide*. Show all work neatly and check your answers. Strive to work through difficulties when possible, making note of any exercises where you need additional help. Remember, even if your instructor assigns homework through *MyMathLab*, you should still write out your work.

 Copyright © 2017 Pearson Education, Inc.

Group Project for Chapter 4

Group members who have cell phone plans should describe the total monthly cost of the plan as follows:

$_____ per month buys _____ minutes.

Additional time costs $_____ per minute.
(For simplicity, ignore other charges.)

a. The group should select any three plans, from "basic" to "premier." For each plan selected, write equations that describe the plan in terms of the total monthly cost, y, for x minutes of use. Compare the plans, two at a time. After how many minutes of use will the costs for the two plans be the same? Solve a linear system to obtain your answer. What will be the cost for each plan? Graph the equations in the same rectangular coordinate system. For any given time of use, the best plan is the one whose graph is lowest at that point.

b. Now compare all three plans. Is one plan always a better deal than the other two? If not, determine the number of minutes of use for which each plan is the better deal.

Copyright © 2017 Pearson Education, Inc.

Getting Ready for the Chapter 4 Test

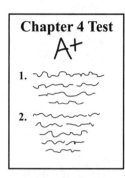

One of the best ways to prepare for a test is to stay on top of your studying, keeping up as your professor proceeds from section to section. Falling behind on one section often makes it difficult to understand the material in the following section. Never wait until the last minute to study for an exam.

Below are several actions that will help you stay organized as you prepare for your test.

How to prepare for your Chapter Test:

☐ **Write down any details that your instructor shares about the test.**
In addition to items such as location, date, time, and essentials to bring, be sure to listen carefully for specific information about the topics covered. Communicate with your instructor concerning any details that may be unclear to you.

☐ **Read the Chapter Summary that begins on page 335 of your textbook.**
Study the appropriate sections in the Chapter Summary. This summary contains the most important material in each section including, definitions, concepts, procedures, and examples.

☐ **Review your *Learning Guide*.**
Go back through the *Solved Problems* and *Pencil Problems* in this chapter of your *Learning Guide*. You may find it helpful to cover up solutions and work through the problems again.

☐ **Study your notes and homework.**
Read through your class notes that you took during this unit, and review the corresponding homework assignments.

☐ **Review quizzes and other feedback from your professor.**
Review any quizzes you have taken and be sure you understand any errors that you made. Seek help with any concepts that are still unclear.

☐ **Complete the Review Exercises that begin on page 337 of your textbook.**
Work the assigned problems from the Review Exercises. These exercises represent the most significant problems for each of the chapter's sections. The answers for all Review Exercises are in the back of your textbook.

☐ **Take the Chapter Test on page 339 of your textbook.**
  • Find a quiet place to take the Chapter Test.
  • Do not use notes, index cards, or any resources other than those your instructor will allow during the actual test.
  • After completing the entire test, check your answers in the back of the textbook.
  • Watch the *Chapter Test Prep Video* to review any exercises you may have missed.

 Copyright © 2017 Pearson Education, Inc.

Chapter 5.R Exponents and Polynomials
Integrated Review

Learning Objectives
   1. Evaluate exponential expressions.

Learning Objective #1: Evaluate exponential expressions.	
✔ *Solved Problem #1*	✎ *Pencil Problem #1* ✎
1a. Evaluate 6^2.	**1a.** Evaluate 9^2.
$6^2 = 6 \cdot 6 = 36$	
1b. Evaluate 2^3.	**1b.** Evaluate 2^5.
$2^3 = 2 \cdot 2 \cdot 2 = 8$	
1c. Evaluate $2 \cdot 7^2$.	**1c.** Evaluate $5 \cdot 3^4$.
$2 \cdot 7^2 = 2 \cdot 7 \cdot 7 = 98$	

Answers for Pencil Problems:

1a. 81   **1b.** 32   **1c.** 405

Copyright © 2017 Pearson Education, Inc.

Section 5.1
Adding and Subtracting Polynomials

What? Me? Racist?

More than 2 million people have tested their racial prejudice using an online version of the Implicit Association Test. Most groups' average scores fall between "slight" and "moderate" bias, but the differences among groups, by age and by political identification, are intriguing. The graph below shows differences among various age groups.

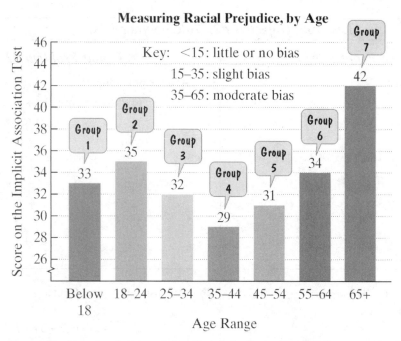

Measuring Racial Prejudice, by Age

Key: <15: little or no bias
15–35: slight bias
35–65: moderate bias

Source: The Race Implicit Association Test on the Project Implicit Demonstration Website

In this section's Exercise Set you will encounter a similar graph that shows bias scores based on political identification and you will work with mathematical models that measure such bias:

First Steps:

☐ **Take comprehensive notes** from your instructor's lecture and insert your notes into this section of the *Learning Guide*. Be sure to write down all examples, definitions, and other key concepts. Additional learning resources include the *Video Lecture Series*, the *PowerPoints*, and Section 5.1 of your textbook which begins on page 342.

☐ Complete the *Concept and Vocabulary Check* on page 348 of the textbook.

Guided Practice:

☐ Review each of the following *Solved Problems* and complete each *Pencil Problem*.

Copyright © 2017 Pearson Education, Inc.

Learning Objective #1: Understand the vocabulary used to describe polynomials.

✔ Solved Problem #1

1. Identify the polynomial as a monomial, a binomial, or a trinomial. Give the degree of the polynomial.

$$7x^5 - 3x^3 + 8$$

$7x^5 - 3x^3 + 8$ is a trinomial of degree 5.

✎ Pencil Problem #1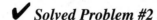

1. Identify the polynomial as a monomial, a binomial, or a trinomial. Give the degree of the polynomial.

$$x^2 - 3x + 4$$

Learning Objective #2: Add polynomials.

✔ Solved Problem #2

2a. Add the polynomials:
$$(-11x^3 + 7x^2 - 11x - 5) + (16x^3 - 3x^2 + 3x - 15)$$

$(-11x^3 + 7x^2 - 11x - 5) + (16x^3 - 3x^2 + 3x - 15)$
$= -11x^3 + 7x^2 - 11x - 5 + 16x^3 - 3x^2 + 3x - 15$
$= -11x^3 + 16x^3 + 7x^2 - 3x^2 - 11x + 3x - 5 - 15$
$= 5x^3 + 4x^2 - 8x - 20$

✎ Pencil Problem #2

2a. Add the polynomials:
$$(4x^2 - 6x + 12) + (x^2 + 3x + 1)$$

2b. Add $-11x^3 + 7x^2 - 11x - 5$ and $16x^3 - 3x^2 + 3x - 15$ using a vertical format.

$-11x^3 + 7x^2 - 11x - 5$
$\underline{+16x^3 - 3x^2 + 3x - 15}$
$\quad 5x^3 + 4x^2 - 8x - 20$

2b. Add using a vertical format:

$$4x^3 - 6x^2 + 5x - 7$$
$$\underline{-9x^3 \qquad\quad -4x + 3}$$

Learning Objective #3: Subtract polynomials.

✔ Solved Problem #3

3a. Subtract $3x^3 - 8x^2 - 5x + 6$ from $10x^3 - 5x^2 + 7x - 2$.

$(10x^3 - 5x^2 + 7x - 2) - (3x^3 - 8x^2 - 5x + 6)$
$= 10x^3 - 5x^2 + 7x - 2 - 3x^3 + 8x^2 + 5x - 6$
$= 10x^3 - 3x^3 - 5x^2 + 8x^2 + 7x + 5x - 2 - 6$
$= 7x^3 + 3x^2 + 12x - 8$

✎ Pencil Problem #3

3a. Subtract $y^2 - 8y + 9$ from $6y^3 + 2y^2 - y - 11$.

Copyright © 2017 Pearson Education, Inc.

3b. Use the method of subtracting in columns to find $(8y^3 - 10y^2 - 14y - 2) - (5y^3 - 3y + 6)$.

$$8y^3 - 10y^2 - 14y - 2$$
$$-\left(5y^3 \qquad -3y + 6\right)$$

To subtract, add the opposite of the polynomial being subtracted.

$$8y^3 - 10y^2 - 14y - 2$$
$$-5y^3 \qquad\quad +3y - 6$$
$$\overline{3y^3 - 10y^2 - 11y - 8}$$

3b. Use a vertical format to subtract the polynomials.

$$7x^3 + 5x^2 - 3$$
$$-\left(-2x^3 - 6x^2 + 5\right)$$

Learning Objective #4:	Graph equations defined by polynomials of degree 2.

✔ *Solved Problem #4*

4. Graph the equation $y = x^2 - 1$.

Make a table of values using integers from -3 to 3.

Table of values.

x	$y = x^2 - 1$	(x, y)
-3	$y = (-3)^2 - 1 = 8$	$(-3, 8)$
-2	$y = (-2)^2 - 1 = 3$	$(-2, 3)$
-1	$y = (-1)^2 - 1 = 0$	$(-1, 0)$
0	$y = (0)^2 - 1 = -1$	$(0, -1)$
1	$y = (1)^2 - 1 = 0$	$(1, 0)$
2	$y = (2)^2 - 1 = 3$	$(2, 3)$
3	$y = (3)^2 - 1 = 8$	$(3, 8)$

✎ *Pencil Problem #4*

4. Graph the equation $y = 4 - x^2$.

Make a table of values using integers from -3 to 3.

Copyright © 2017 Pearson Education, Inc.

Plot the points and connect them with a smooth curve.

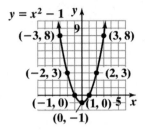

Answers for Pencil Problems *(Textbook Exercise references in parentheses)*:

1. trinomial of degree 2   *(5.1 #9)*

2a. $5x^2 - 3x + 13$ *(5.1 #23)*   **2b.** $-5x^3 - 6x^2 + x - 4$ *(5.1 #47)*

3a. $6y^3 + y^2 + 7y - 20$ *(5.1 #65)*   **3b.** $9x^3 + 11x^2 - 8$ *(5.1 #81)*

4.

x	$y = 4 - x^2$	(x, y)
-3	$y = 4 - (-3)^2 = -5$	$(-3, -5)$
-2	$y = 4 - (-2)^2 = 0$	$(-2, 0)$
-1	$y = 4 - (-1)^2 = 3$	$(-1, 3)$
0	$y = 4 - (0)^2 = 4$	$(0, 4)$
1	$y = 4 - (1)^2 = 3$	$(1, 3)$
2	$y = 4 - (2)^2 = 0$	$(2, 0)$
3	$y = 4 - (3)^2 = -5$	$(3, -5)$

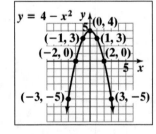

(5.1 #93)

Homework:

☐ **Review the Section 5.1 summary** on page 411 of the textbook.

☐ **Insert your homework** into this section of the *Learning Guide*. Show all work neatly and check your answers. Strive to work through difficulties when possible, making note of any exercises where you need additional help. Remember, even if your instructor assigns homework through *MyMathLab*, you should still write out your work.

          Copyright © 2017 Pearson Education, Inc.

Section 5.2
Multiplying Polynomials

It's all Greek to me!

As discussed earlier in the textbook, the ancient Greeks believed that the most visually pleasing rectangles have a ratio of length to width of approximately 1.618 to 1.

With the exception of the squares on the lower left and the upper right, the interior of this geometric figure is filled entirely with these golden rectangles. Furthermore, the large rectangle is also a golden rectangle.

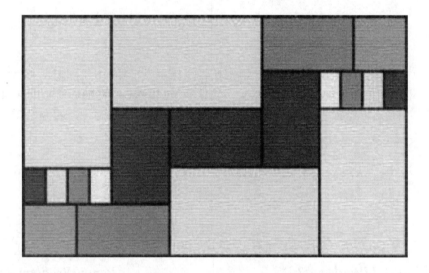

The total area of the large rectangle can be found in many ways. This is because the area of any large rectangular region is related to the areas of the smaller rectangles that make up that region.

In this section, we apply areas of rectangles as a way to picture the multiplication of polynomials.

First Steps:

☐ **Take comprehensive notes** from your instructor's lecture and insert your notes into this section of the *Learning Guide*. Be sure to write down all examples, definitions, and other key concepts. Additional learning resources include the *Video Lecture Series*, the *PowerPoints*, and Section 5.2 of your textbook which begins on page 351.

☐ Complete the *Concept and Vocabulary Check* on page 358 of the textbook.

Guided Practice:

☐ Review each of the following *Solved Problems* and complete each *Pencil Problem*.

Learning Objective #1: Use the product rule for exponents.	
✔ **Solved Problem #1**	✎ **Pencil Problem #1** 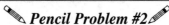
1a. Multiply the expression using the product rule. $$2^2 \cdot 2^4$$ $2^2 \cdot 2^4 = 2^{2+4}$ $\quad = 2^6$ or 64	**1a.** Multiply the expression using the product rule. $$x^{15} \cdot x^3$$
1b. Multiply the expression using the product rule. $$y^4 \cdot y^3 \cdot y^2$$ $y^4 \cdot y^3 \cdot y^2 = y^{4+3+2}$ $\quad = y^9$	**1b.** Multiply the expression using the product rule. $$x^2 \cdot x^6 \cdot x^3$$

Learning Objective #2: Use the power rule for exponents.	
✔ **Solved Problem #2**	✎ **Pencil Problem #2**
2a. Simplify the expression using the power rule. $$\left(x^9\right)^{10}$$ $\left(x^9\right)^{10} = x^{9 \cdot 10}$ $\quad = x^{90}$	**2a.** Simplify the expression using the power rule. $$\left(x^{15}\right)^3$$
2b. Simplify the expression using the power rule. $$\left[(-5)^7\right]^3$$ $\left[(-5)^7\right]^3 = (-5)^{7 \cdot 3}$ $\quad = (-5)^{21}$	**2b.** Simplify the expression using the power rule. $$\left[(-20)^3\right]^3$$

Copyright © 2017 Pearson Education, Inc.

Learning Objective #3: Use the products-to-powers rule.	
✔ **Solved Problem #3**	✎ **Pencil Problem #3**✎
3a. Simplify the expression using the powers-to-products rule. $$(2x)^4$$ $$(2x)^4 = 2^4 x^4$$ $$= 16x^4$$	**3a.** Simplify the expression using the powers-to-products rule. $$(-5x)^2$$
3b. Simplify the expression using the powers-to-products rule. $$\left(-4y^2\right)^3$$ $$\left(-4y^2\right)^3 = (-4)^3 \left(y^2\right)^3$$ $$= (-4)^3 y^{2\cdot3}$$ $$= -64y^6$$	**3b.** Simplify the expression using the powers-to-products rule. $$\left(-2y^6\right)^4$$

Learning Objective #4: Multiply monomials.	
✔ **Solved Problem #4**	✎ **Pencil Problem #4**✎
4. Multiply: $(-5x^4)(4x^5)$ $$(-5x^4)(4x^5) = (-5\cdot4)(x^4 \cdot x^5)$$ $$= -20x^9$$	**4.** Multiply: $(2x^2)(-3x)(8x^4)$

Learning Objective #5: Multiply a monomial and a polynomial.

✔ *Solved Problem #5*	✎ *Pencil Problem #5*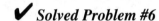

5. Multiply: $6x^2(5x^3 - 2x + 3)$

$$6x^2(5x^3 - 2x + 3) = 6x^2 \cdot 5x^3 - 6x^2 \cdot 2x + 6x^2 \cdot 3$$
$$= 30x^5 - 12x^3 + 18x^2$$

5. Multiply: $-3x^2(-4x^2 + x - 5)$

Learning Objective #6: Multiply polynomials when neither is a monomial.

✔ *Solved Problem #6*	✎ *Pencil Problem #6*✎

6. Multiply: $(5x + 3)(2x - 7)$

$$(5x + 3)(2x - 7) = 10x^2 - 35x + 6x - 21$$
$$= 10x^2 - 29x - 21$$

6. Multiply: $(2x - 5)(x + 4)$

Answers for Pencil Problems *(Textbook Exercise references in parentheses)*:

1a. x^{18} *(5.2 #1)*   **1b.** x^{11} *(5.2 #5)*   **2a.** x^{45} *(5.2 #11)*   **2b.** $(-20)^9$ *(5.2 #13)*

3a. $25x^2$ *(5.2 #17)*   **3b.** $16y^{24}$ *(5.2 #21)*

4. $-48x^7$ *(5.2 #33)*   **5.** $12x^4 - 3x^3 + 15x^2$ *(5.2 #53)*   **6.** $2x^2 + 3x - 20$ *(5.2 #63)*

Homework:

☐ **Review the Section 5.2 summary** on page 412 of the textbook.

☐ **Insert your homework** into this section of the *Learning Guide*. Show all work neatly and check your answers. Strive to work through difficulties when possible, making note of any exercises where you need additional help. Remember, even if your instructor assigns homework through *MyMathLab*, you should still write out your work.

Copyright © 2017 Pearson Education, Inc.

Built for *SPEED!*

After working through the previous section, students often wonder if there are fast methods for finding products of polynomials.
Fortunately, the answer is "yes."

In this section of the textbook, we will use the distributive property to develop patterns that will let you multiply certain binomials quite rapidly.

First Steps:

☐ **Take comprehensive notes** from your instructor's lecture and insert your notes into this section of the *Learning Guide*. Be sure to write down all examples, definitions, and other key concepts. Additional learning resources include the *Video Lecture Series*, the *PowerPoints*, and Section 5.3 of your textbook which begins on page 361.

☐ Complete the **Concept and Vocabulary Check** on page 367 of the textbook.

Guided Practice:

☐ Review each of the following **Solved Problems** and complete each **Pencil Problem**.

Learning Objective #1: Use FOIL in polynomial multiplication.	
✔ *Solved Problem #1*	✎ *Pencil Problem #1*✎
1a. Multiply: $(x+5)(x+6)$	**1a.** Multiply: $(y-7)(y+3)$

$$(x+5)(x+6) = \overset{F}{\overbrace{x \cdot x}} + \overset{O}{\overbrace{6 \cdot x}} + \overset{I}{\overbrace{5 \cdot x}} + \overset{L}{\overbrace{5 \cdot 6}}$$
$$= x^2 + 6x + 5x + 30$$
$$= x^2 + 11x + 30$$

1b. Multiply: $(7x+5)(4x-3)$	**1b.** Multiply: $(2x-3)(5x+3)$

$$(7x+5)(4x-3) = \overset{F}{\overbrace{7x \cdot 4x}} + \overset{O}{\overbrace{7x(-3)}} + \overset{I}{\overbrace{5 \cdot 4x}} + \overset{L}{\overbrace{5(-3)}}$$
$$= 28x^2 - 21x + 20x - 15$$
$$= 28x^2 - x - 15$$

Learning Objective #2: Multiply the sum and difference of two terms.

✔ **Solved Problem #2**	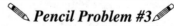 **Pencil Problem #2**

2a. Multiply: $(7y+8)(7y-8)$

Since this product is of the form $(A+B)(A-B)$, use the special–product formula

$(A+B)(A-B) = A^2 - B^2$.

$$\underset{\substack{\text{first term} \\ \text{squared}}}{\quad} \underset{\substack{\text{second term} \\ \text{squared}}}{\quad}$$

$$(7y+8)(7y-8) = (7y)^2 - 8^2$$
$$= 49y^2 - 64$$

2a. Multiply: $(3x+2)(3x-2)$

2b. Multiply: $(2a^3+3)(2a^3-3)$

Since this product is of the form $(A+B)(A-B)$, use the special–product formula

$(A+B)(A-B) = A^2 - B^2$.

$$\underset{\substack{\text{first term} \\ \text{squared}}}{\quad} \underset{\substack{\text{second term} \\ \text{squared}}}{\quad}$$

$$(2a^3+3)(2a^3-3) = (2a^3)^2 - 3^2$$
$$= 4a^6 - 9$$

2b. Multiply: $(x^{10}+5)(x^{10}-5)$

Learning Objective #3: Find the square of a binomial sum.

✔ **Solved Problem #3**	**Pencil Problem #3**

3a. Multiply: $(x+10)^2$

Use the special-product formula
$(A+B)^2 = A^2 + 2AB + B^2$.

$$\underset{\substack{\text{first term} \\ \text{squared}}}{\quad} \underset{\substack{2 \cdot \text{product} \\ \text{of the terms}}}{\quad} \underset{\substack{\text{last term} \\ \text{squared}}}{\quad}$$

$$(x+10)^2 = x^2 + 2 \cdot 10x + 10^2$$
$$= x^2 + 20x + 100$$

3a. Multiply: $(x+2)^2$

Copyright © 2017 Pearson Education, Inc.

3b. Multiply: $(5x+4)^2$

Use the special-product formula
$(A+B)^2 = A^2 + 2AB + B^2$.

$$(5x+4)^2 = \overbrace{(5x)^2}^{\substack{\text{first term}\\\text{squared}}} + \overbrace{2\cdot 20x}^{\substack{2\cdot\text{product}\\\text{of the terms}}} + \overbrace{4^2}^{\substack{\text{last term}\\\text{squared}}}$$
$$= 25x^2 + 40x + 16$$

3b. Multiply: $(x^8 + 3)^2$

Learning Objective #4: Find the square of a binomial difference.

✔ *Solved Problem #4*

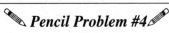 *Pencil Problem #4*

4a. Multiply: $(x-9)^2$

Use the special-product formula
$(A-B)^2 = A^2 - 2AB + B^2$.

$$(x-9)^2 = \overbrace{x^2}^{\substack{\text{first term}\\\text{squared}}} - \overbrace{2\cdot 9x}^{\substack{2\cdot\text{product}\\\text{of the terms}}} + \overbrace{9^2}^{\substack{\text{last term}\\\text{squared}}}$$
$$= x^2 - 18x + 81$$

4a. Multiply: $(x-3)^2$

4b. Multiply: $(7x-3)^2$

Use the special-product formula
$(A-B)^2 = A^2 - 2AB + B^2$.

$$(7x-3)^2 = \overbrace{(7x)^2}^{\substack{\text{first term}\\\text{squared}}} - \overbrace{2\cdot 21x}^{\substack{2\cdot\text{product}\\\text{of the terms}}} + \overbrace{3^2}^{\substack{\text{last term}\\\text{squared}}}$$
$$= 49x^2 - 42x + 9$$

4b. Multiply: $(7-2x)^2$

Copyright © 2017 Pearson Education, Inc.

Answers for Pencil Problems *(Textbook Exercise references in parentheses)*:

1a. $y^2 - 4y - 21$ *(5.3 #3)*

1b. $10x^2 - 9x - 9$ *(5.3 #9)*

2a. $9x^2 - 4$ *(5.3 #27)*

2b. $x^{20} - 25$ *(5.3 #43)*

3a. $x^2 + 4x + 4$ *(5.3 #45)*

3b. $x^{16} + 6x^8 + 9$ *(5.3 #61)*

4a. $x^2 - 6x + 9$ *(5.3 #49)*

4b. $49 - 28x + 4x^2$ *(5.3 #55)*

Homework:

☐ **Review the Section 5.3 summary** on page 412 of the textbook.

☐ **Insert your homework** into this section of the *Learning Guide*. Show all work neatly and check your answers. Strive to work through difficulties when possible, making note of any exercises where you need additional help. Remember, even if your instructor assigns homework through *MyMathLab*, you should still write out your work.

Copyright © 2017 Pearson Education, Inc.

Section 5.4
Polynomials in Several Variables

Timber !!!!

The next time you visit a lumberyard and go rummaging through piles of wood, think polynomials!

But these polynomials are a bit different from those we have encountered so far.

In this section of the textbook, we will explore a polynomial in two variables that the construction industry uses to determine the number of board feet that can be manufactured from a tree with a diameter of x inches and a length of y feet.

First Steps:

☐ **Take comprehensive notes** from your instructor's lecture and insert your notes into this section of the *Learning Guide*. Be sure to write down all examples, definitions, and other key concepts. Additional learning resources include the *Video Lecture Series*, the *PowerPoints*, and Section 5.4 of your textbook which begins on page 370.

☐ Complete the *Concept and Vocabulary Check* on page 375 of the textbook.

Guided Practice:

☐ Review each of the following *Solved Problems* and complete each *Pencil Problem*.

Learning Objective #1: Evaluate polynomials in several variables.

✔ *Solved Problem #1*	✎ *Pencil Problem #1* ✎
1. Evaluate $3x^3y + xy^2 + 5y + 6$ for $x = -1$ and $y = 5$.	**1.** Evaluate $2x^2y - 5y + 3$ for $x = 2$ and $y = -3$.

Begin by substituting -1 in for x and 5 in for y.

$$\begin{aligned} 3x^3y + xy^2 + 5y + 6 &= 3(-1)^3(5) + (-1)(5)^2 + 5(5) + 6 \\ &= 3(-1)(5) + (-1)(25) + 5(5) + 6 \\ &= -15 - 25 + 25 + 6 \\ &= -9 \end{aligned}$$

Copyright © 2017 Pearson Education, Inc.

Learning Objective #2: Understand the vocabulary of polynomials in two variables.

✔ **Solved Problem #2**

2. Determine the coefficient of each term, the degree of each term, and the degree of the polynomial:

$$8x^4y^5 - 7x^3y^2 - x^2y - 5x + 11$$

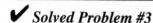

Term Term Term Term Term
$8x^4y^5$ $-7x^3y^2$ $-x^2y$ $-5x$ $+11$

Term	Coefficient	Degree
$8x^4y^5$	8	$4+5=9$
$-7x^3y^2$	-7	$3+2=5$
$-x^2y$	-1	$2+1=3$
$-5x$	-5	1
11	11	0

The degree of the polynomial is the highest degree of all its terms, which is 9.

✏ **Pencil Problem #2** ✏

2. Determine the coefficient of each term, the degree of each term, and the degree of the polynomial:

$$x^3y^2 - 5x^2y^7 + 6y^2 - 3$$

Learning Objective #3: Add and subtract polynomials in several variables.

✔ **Solved Problem #3**

3a. Add: $(-8x^2y - 3xy + 6) + (10x^2y + 5xy - 10)$

$(-8x^2y - 3xy + 6) + (10x^2y + 5xy - 10)$
$= -8x^2y - 3xy + 6 + 10x^2y + 5xy - 10$
$= -8x^2y + 10x^2y - 3xy + 5xy + 6 - 10$
$= 2x^2y + 2xy - 4$

✏ **Pencil Problem #3** ✏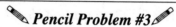

3a. Add: $(4x^2y + 8xy + 11) + (-2x^2y + 5xy + 2)$

3b. Subtract:
$(7x^3 - 10x^2y + 2xy^2 - 5) - (4x^3 - 12x^2y - 3xy^2 + 5)$

$(7x^3 - 10x^2y + 2xy^2 - 5) - (4x^3 - 12x^2y - 3xy^2 + 5)$
$= 7x^3 - 10x^2y + 2xy^2 - 5 - 4x^3 + 12x^2y + 3xy^2 - 5$
$= 7x^3 - 4x^3 - 10x^2y + 12x^2y + 2xy^2 + 3xy^2 - 5 - 5$
$= 3x^3 + 2x^2y + 5xy^2 - 10$

3b. Subtract: $(x^3 + 7xy - 5y^2) - (6x^3 - xy + 4y^2)$

Copyright © 2017 Pearson Education, Inc.

Learning Objective #4: Multiply polynomials in several variables.	
✔ *Solved Problem #4*	✎ *Pencil Problem #4* ✎
4a. Multiply: $(6xy^3)(10x^4y^2)$	**4a.** Multiply: $(-8x^3y^4)(3x^2y^5)$

$$(6xy^3)(10x^4y^2) = (6 \cdot 10)(x \cdot x^4)(y^3 \cdot y^2)$$
$$= 60x^{1+4}y^{3+2}$$
$$= 60x^5y^5$$

4b. Multiply: $6xy^2(10x^4y^5 - 2x^2y + 3)$	**4b.** Multiply: $4ab^2(7a^2b^3 + 2ab)$

$$6xy^2(10x^4y^5 - 2x^2y + 3)$$
$$= 6xy^2 \cdot 10x^4y^5 - 6xy^2 \cdot 2x^2y + 6xy^2 \cdot 3$$
$$= 60x^{1+4}y^{2+5} - 12x^{1+2}y^{2+1} + 18xy^2$$
$$= 60x^5y^7 - 12x^3y^3 + 18xy^2$$

4c. Multiply: $(7x - 6y)(3x - y)$	**4c.** Multiply: $(x - 3y)(2x + 7y)$

$$(7x - 6y)(3x - y)$$
$$= \overbrace{(7x)(3x)}^{F} + \overbrace{(7x)(-y)}^{O} + \overbrace{(-6y)(3x)}^{I} + \overbrace{(-6y)(-y)}^{L}$$
$$= 21x^2 - 7xy - 18xy + 6y^2$$
$$= 21x^2 - 25xy + 6y^2$$

Copyright © 2017 Pearson Education, Inc.

4d. Multiply: $(6xy^2 + 5x)(6xy^2 - 5x)$

$$\overbrace{(6xy^2 + 5x)(6xy^2 - 5x)}^{(A+B)(A-B)} = \overbrace{(6xy^2)^2}^{A^2} - \overbrace{(5x)^2}^{B^2}$$
$$= 36x^2y^4 - 25x^2$$

4d. Multiply: $(x^2 - 2y^2)^2$

Answers for Pencil Problems *(Textbook Exercise references in parentheses)*:

1. -6 *(5.4 #5)*

2.

Term	Coefficient	Degree
x^3y^2	1	$3+2=5$
$-5x^2y^7$	-5	$2+7=9$
$6y^2$	6	2
-3	-3	0

The degree of the polynomial is 9. *(5.4 #7)*

3a. $2x^2y + 13xy + 13$ *(5.4 #11)*   **3b.** $-5x^3 + 8xy - 9y^2$ *(5.4 #15)*

4a. $-24x^5y^9$ *(5.4 #29)*   **4b.** $28a^3b^5 + 8a^2b^3$ *(5.4 #35)*

4c. $2x^2 + xy - 21y^2$ *(5.4 #41)*   **4d.** $x^4 - 4x^2y^2 + 4y^4$ *(5.4 #51)*

Homework:

☐ **Review the Section 5.4 summary** which begins on page 412 of the textbook.

☐ **Insert your homework** into this section of the *Learning Guide*. Show all work neatly and check your answers. Strive to work through difficulties when possible, making note of any exercises where you need additional help. Remember, even if your instructor assigns homework through *MyMathLab*, you should still write out your work.

Copyright © 2017 Pearson Education, Inc.

Section 5.5
Dividing Polynomials

Have you seen the latest blockbuster?

As individuals and as a nation, we've grown up with movies. Our images of love, war, family, country, and even the things that terrify us, have been greatly influenced by what we've seen on the big screen.

In this section's Exercise Set, we'll model our love for movies with polynomials and polynomial division.

First Steps:

☐ **Take comprehensive notes** from your instructor's lecture and insert your notes into this section of the *Learning Guide*. Be sure to write down all examples, definitions, and other key concepts. Additional learning resources include the *Video Lecture Series*, the *PowerPoints*, and Section 5.5 of your textbook which begins on page 379.

☐ Complete the *Concept and Vocabulary Check* on page 385 of the textbook.

Guided Practice:

☐ Review each of the following *Solved Problems* and complete each *Pencil Problem*.

Learning Objective #1: Use the quotient rule for exponents.	
✔ *Solved Problem #1*	✎ *Pencil Problem #1* ✎
1a. Divide the expression using the quotient rule: $\dfrac{5^{12}}{5^4}$	**1a.** Divide the expression using the quotient rule: $\dfrac{3^{20}}{3^5}$
$\dfrac{5^{12}}{5^4} = 5^{12-4}$ $\qquad = 5^8$	
1b. Divide the expression using the quotient rule: $\dfrac{x^9}{x^2}$	**1b.** Divide the expression using the quotient rule: $\dfrac{x^6}{x^2}$
$\dfrac{x^9}{x^2} = x^{9-2}$ $\qquad = x^7$	

Learning Objective #2: Use the zero-exponent rule.	
✔ *Solved Problem #2*	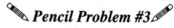 *Pencil Problem #2*

2a. Use the zero-exponent rule to simplify the expression: 14^0

The zero-exponent rule states that if b is any real number other than 0, then $b^0 = 1$.

Thus, $14^0 = 1$.

2a. Use the zero-exponent rule to simplify the expression: $(-2)^0$

2b. Use the zero-exponent rule to simplify the expression: -10^0

Note that only the 10 is raised to the 0 power.

$$-10^0 = -1 \cdot 10^0$$
$$= -1 \cdot 1$$
$$= -1$$

2b. Use the zero-exponent rule to simplify the expression: -2^0

2c. Use the zero-exponent rule to simplify the expression: $20x^0$

Note that only the x is raised to the 0 power.

$$20x^0 = 20 \cdot 1$$
$$= 20$$

2c. Use the zero-exponent rule to simplify the expression: $(100y)^0$

Learning Objective #3: Use the quotients-to-powers rule.	
✔ *Solved Problem #3*	✎ *Pencil Problem #3*

3a. Simplify the expression using the quotients-to-powers rule: $\left(\dfrac{x}{5}\right)^2$

$$\left(\frac{x}{5}\right)^2 = \frac{x^2}{5^2}$$
$$= \frac{x^2}{25}$$

3a. Simplify the expression using the quotients-to-powers rule: $\left(\dfrac{x^2}{4}\right)^3$

 Copyright © 2017 Pearson Education, Inc.

3b. Simplify the expression using the quotients-to-powers rule: $\left(\dfrac{2a^{10}}{b^3}\right)^4$

$$\left(\frac{2a^{10}}{b^3}\right)^4 = \frac{2^4(a^{10})^4}{(b^3)^4}$$

$$= \frac{16a^{40}}{b^{12}}$$

3b. Simplify the expression using the quotients-to-powers rule: $\left(\dfrac{-2a^7}{b^4}\right)^5$

Learning Objective #4: Divide monomials.

✔ Solved Problem #4

4a. Divide: $\dfrac{3x^4}{15x^4}$

$$\frac{3x^4}{15x^4} = \frac{3}{15}x^{4-4}$$

$$= \frac{1}{5}x^0$$

$$= \frac{1}{5}$$

✎ Pencil Problem #4 ✎

4a. Divide: $\dfrac{30x^{10}}{10x^5}$

4b. Divide: $\dfrac{9x^6y^5}{3xy^2}$

$$\frac{9x^6y^5}{3xy^2} = \frac{9}{3}\cdot x^{6-1}y^{5-2}$$

$$= 3x^5y^3$$

4b. Divide: $\dfrac{-18x^{14}y^2}{36x^2y^2}$

Learning Objective #5: Check polynomial division.

✔ Solved Problem #5

5. Check your answer to 4b by showing that the product of the divisor and the quotient is the dividend.

$$(3xy^2)(3x^5y^3) = 3\cdot 3\cdot x^{1+5}\cdot y^{2+3}$$

$$= 9x^6y^5$$

✎ Pencil Problem #5 ✎

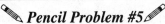

5. Check your answer to 4b by showing that the product of the divisor and the quotient is the dividend.

Copyright © 2017 Pearson Education, Inc.

Learning Objective #6: Divide a polynomial by a monomial.	
✔ *Solved Problem #6*	✎ *Pencil Problem #6*✎

6a. Divide: $\dfrac{-15x^9 + 6x^5 - 9x^3}{3x^2}$

$$\frac{-15x^9 + 6x^5 - 9x^3}{3x^2} = \frac{-15x^9}{3x^2} + \frac{6x^5}{3x^2} - \frac{9x^3}{3x^2}$$
$$= -5x^7 + 2x^3 - 3x$$

6a. Divide: $\dfrac{18x^5 + 6x^4 + 9x^3}{3x^2}$

6b. Divide: $\dfrac{18x^7 y^6 - 6x^2 y^3 + 60xy^2}{6xy^2}$

$$\frac{18x^7 y^6 - 6x^2 y^3 + 60xy^2}{6xy^2} = \frac{18x^7 y^6}{6xy^2} - \frac{6x^2 y^3}{6xy^2} + \frac{60xy^2}{6xy^2}$$
$$= 3x^6 y^4 - xy + 10$$

6b. Divide: $\dfrac{12x^2 y^2 + 6x^2 y - 15xy^2}{3xy}$

Answers for Pencil Problems *(Textbook Exercise references in parentheses)*:

1a. 3^{15} *(5.5 #1)* **1b.** x^4 *(5.5 #3)* **2a.** 1 *(5.5 #13)* **2b.** -1 *(5.5 #15)* **2c.** 1 *(5.5 #19)*

3a. $\dfrac{x^6}{64}$ *(5.5 #27)* **3b.** $-\dfrac{32a^{35}}{b^{20}}$ *(5.5 #33)* **4a.** $3x^5$ *(5.5 #37)* **4b.** $-\dfrac{1}{2}x^{12}$ *(5.5 #47)*

5. $\left(-\dfrac{1}{2}x^{12}\right)\left(36x^2 y^2\right) = -18x^{14}y^2$ *(5.5 #47)* **6a.** $6x^3 + 2x^2 + 3x$ *(5.5 #61)* **6b.** $4xy + 2x - 5y$ *(5.5 #75)*

Homework:

☐ **Review the Section 5.5 summary** on page 413 of the textbook.

☐ **Insert your homework** into this section of the *Learning Guide*. Show all work neatly and check your answers. Strive to work through difficulties when possible, making note of any exercises where you need additional help. Remember, even if your instructor assigns homework through *MyMathLab*, you should still write out your work.

 Copyright © 2017 Pearson Education, Inc.

Are You Having a Déjà Vu?

In this section of the textbook, we will study the process for dividing a polynomial by a binomial. This process may remind you of long division of whole numbers.

Let's review long division of whole numbers by dividing 3983 by 26.

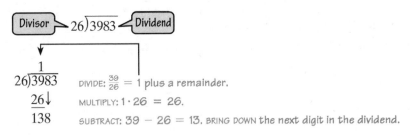

$$26\overline{)3983}$$

Divisor — $26\overline{)3983}$ — Dividend

$$
\begin{array}{r}
1 \\
26\overline{)3983} \\
26\downarrow \\
\hline
138
\end{array}
$$

DIVIDE: $\frac{39}{26} = 1$ plus a remainder.

MULTIPLY: $1 \cdot 26 = 26$.

SUBTRACT: $39 - 26 = 13$. BRING DOWN the next digit in the dividend.

$$
\begin{array}{r}
15 \\
26\overline{)3983} \\
26 \\
\hline
138 \\
130 \\
\hline
83
\end{array}
$$

DIVIDE: $\frac{138}{26} = 5$ plus a remainder.

MULTIPLY: $5 \cdot 26 = 130$.

SUBTRACT: $138 - 130 = 8$. BRING DOWN the next digit in the dividend.

$$
\begin{array}{r}
153 \\
26\overline{)3983} \\
26 \\
\hline
138 \\
130 \\
\hline
83 \\
78 \\
\hline
5
\end{array}
$$

DIVIDE: $\frac{83}{26} = 3$ plus a remainder.

MULTIPLY: $3 \cdot 26 = 78$.

SUBTRACT: $83 - 78 = 5$. There are no more digits to bring down, so the remainder is 5.

The quotient is 153 and the remainder is 5. This can be written as $153\frac{5}{26}$.

First Steps:

☐ **Take comprehensive notes** from your instructor's lecture and insert your notes into this section of the *Learning Guide*. Be sure to write down all examples, definitions, and other key concepts. Additional learning resources include the *Video Lecture Series*, the *PowerPoints*, and Section 5.6 of your textbook which begins on page 388.

☐ Complete the *Concept and Vocabulary Check* on page 395 of the textbook.

Copyright © 2017 Pearson Education, Inc.

Guided Practice:

☐ Review each of the following *Solved Problems* and complete each *Pencil Problem*.

Learning Objective #1: Divide polynomials by binomials.

✔ Solved Problem #1

1a. Divide $x^2 + 14x + 45$ by $x + 9$.

Arrange the terms in the dividend, $x^2 + 14x + 45$, and the divisor, $x + 9$, in descending order.

$$x + 9 \overline{) x^2 + 14x + 45}$$

Divide x^2 by x: $\dfrac{x^2}{x} = x$. Align like terms.

$$\begin{array}{r} x \\ x + 9 \overline{) x^2 + 14x + 45} \end{array}$$

Multiply each term in the divisor, $x + 9$, by x.

$$\begin{array}{r} x \\ x + 9 \overline{) x^2 + 14x + 45} \\ \underline{x^2 + 9x} \end{array}$$

Subtract $x^2 + 9x$ from $x^2 + 14x$ and bring down the 45.

$$\begin{array}{r} x \\ x + 9 \overline{) x^2 + 14x + 45} \\ \underline{x^2 + 9x} \\ 5x + 45 \end{array}$$

Divide $5x$ by x: $\dfrac{5x}{x} = 5$. Next, multiply each term in the divisor by 5, and then subtract.

$$\begin{array}{r} x + 5 \\ x + 9 \overline{) x^2 + 14x + 45} \\ \underline{x^2 + 9x} \\ 5x + 45 \\ \underline{5x + 45} \\ 0 \end{array}$$

The quotient is $x + 5$ and the remainder is 0.

Thus, $\dfrac{x^2 + 14x + 45}{x + 9} = x + 5$.

✎ Pencil Problem #1 ✎

1a. Divide $x^2 - 5x + 6$ by $x - 3$.

Copyright © 2017 Pearson Education, Inc.

1b. Divide: $\dfrac{6x+8x^2-12}{2x+3}$

Arrange the terms in the numerator (dividend), in descending order:

$$\frac{6x+8x^2-12}{2x+3}=\frac{8x^2+6x-12}{2x+3}$$

$$\begin{array}{r} 4x-3 \\ 2x+3\overline{)8x^2+6x-12} \\ \underline{8x^2+12x} \\ -6x-12 \\ \underline{-6x-9} \\ -3 \end{array}$$

Write your answer in the following format:

$$\frac{\text{Dividend}}{\text{Divisor}}=\text{Quotient}+\frac{\text{Remainder}}{\text{Divisor}}$$

Thus,

$$\frac{6x+8x^2-12}{2x+3}=\overset{\text{Quotient}}{\overbrace{4x-3}}-\frac{\overset{\text{Remainder}}{\overbrace{3}}}{\underbrace{2x+3}_{\text{Divisor}}}$$

$$=4x-3-\frac{3}{2x+3}$$

1b. Divide: $\dfrac{5y+10+y^2}{y+2}$

1c. Divide: $\dfrac{x^3 - 1}{x - 1}$

1c. Divide: $\dfrac{y^4 - 2y^2 + 5}{y - 1}$

Rewrite $x^3 - 1$ using coefficients of 0 on the missing terms gives $x^3 + 0x^2 + 0x - 1$.

$$
\begin{array}{r}
x^2 + x + 1 \\
x-1\overline{\smash{\big)}\,x^3 + 0x^2 + 0x - 1} \\
\underline{x^3 - x^2} \\
x^2 + 0x \\
\underline{x^2 - x} \\
x - 1 \\
\underline{x - 1} \\
0
\end{array}
$$

The quotient is $x^2 + x + 1$ and the remainder is 0.

Thus,

$$\dfrac{x^3 - 1}{x - 1} = x^2 + x + 1$$

Answers for Pencil Problems *(Textbook Exercise references in parentheses)*:

1a. $x - 2$ *(5.6 #5)*

1b. $y + 3 + \dfrac{4}{y + 2}$ *(5.6 #11)*

1c. $y^3 + y^2 - y - 1 + \dfrac{4}{y - 1}$ *(5.6 #35)*

Homework:

☐ **Review the Section 5.6 summary** on page 413 of the textbook.

☐ **Insert your homework** into this section of the *Learning Guide*. Show all work neatly and check your answers. Strive to work through difficulties when possible, making note of any exercises where you need additional help. Remember, even if your instructor assigns homework through *MyMathLab*, you should still write out your work.

   Copyright © 2017 Pearson Education, Inc.

Section 5.7
Negative Exponents and Scientific Notation

What is YOUR Share of the National Debt?

In a recent year there was a budget deficit of about $1,350,000,000,000
and there were approximately 307,000,000 Americans.

In this section of the textbook, we will use exponents and scientific notation to explore
these values, and calculate each citizens' share of the national debt.

First Steps:

☐ **Take comprehensive notes** from your instructor's lecture and insert your notes into this
section of the *Learning Guide*. Be sure to write down all examples, definitions, and other
key concepts. Additional learning resources include the *Video Lecture Series*, the
PowerPoints, and Section 5.7 of your textbook which begins on page 398.

☐ Complete the *Concept and Vocabulary Check* on page 408 of the textbook.

Guided Practice:

☐ Review each of the following *Solved Problems* and complete each *Pencil Problem*.

Learning Objective #1: Use the negative exponent rule.	
✔ *Solved Problem #1*	✎ *Pencil Problem #1* ✎
1a. Use the negative exponent rule to write 5^{-3} with a positive exponent and then simplify.	**1a.** Use the negative exponent rule to write 8^{-2} with a positive exponent and then simplify.
$5^{-3} = \dfrac{1}{5^3}$ $= \dfrac{1}{125}$	
1b. Use the negative exponent rule to write $(-3)^{-4}$ with a positive exponent and then simplify.	**1b.** Use the negative exponent rule to write $(-6)^{-2}$ with a positive exponent and then simplify.
$(-3)^{-4} = \dfrac{1}{(-3)^4}$ $= \dfrac{1}{81}$	

Copyright © 2017 Pearson Education, Inc.

1c. Use the negative exponent rule to write 8^{-1} with a positive exponent and then simplify.

$$8^{-1} = \frac{1}{8^1}$$
$$= \frac{1}{8}$$

1c. Use the negative exponent rule to write -6^{-2} with a positive exponent and then simplify.

1d. Write $\left(\frac{4}{5}\right)^{-2}$ with positive exponents only.

Then simplify, if possible.

$$\left(\frac{4}{5}\right)^{-2} = \frac{5^2}{4^2}$$
$$= \frac{25}{16}$$

1d. Write $\left(\frac{1}{4}\right)^{-2}$ with positive exponents only.

Then simplify, if possible.

1e. Write $\frac{1}{7y^{-2}}$ with positive exponents only.

Then simplify, if possible.

$$\frac{1}{7y^{-2}} = \frac{y^2}{7}$$

1e. Write $\frac{1}{6x^{-5}}$ with positive exponents only.

Then simplify, if possible.

1f. Write $\frac{x^{-1}}{y^{-8}}$ with positive exponents only.

Then simplify, if possible.

$$\frac{x^{-1}}{y^{-8}} = \frac{y^8}{x^1}$$
$$= \frac{y^8}{x}$$

1f. Write $\frac{x^{-8}}{y^{-1}}$ with positive exponents only.

Then simplify, if possible.

Copyright © 2017 Pearson Education, Inc.

Learning Objective #2: Simplify exponential expressions.	
✔ *Solved Problem #2*	✎ *Pencil Problem #2* ✎

2a. Simplify: $x^{-12} \cdot x^2$

$$x^{-12} \cdot x^2 = x^{-12+2}$$
$$= x^{-10}$$
$$= \frac{1}{x^{10}}$$

2a. Simplify: $x^{-8} \cdot x^3$

2b. Simplify: $\dfrac{75x^3}{5x^9}$

$$\frac{75x^3}{5x^9} = \frac{75}{5} \cdot \frac{x^3}{x^9}$$
$$= 15x^{3-9}$$
$$= 15x^{-6}$$
$$= \frac{15}{x^6}$$

2b. Simplify: $\dfrac{30z^5}{10z^{10}}$

2c. Simplify: $\dfrac{(6x^4)^2}{x^{11}}$

$$\frac{(6x^4)^2}{x^{11}} = \frac{6^2(x^4)^2}{x^{11}}$$
$$= \frac{36x^{4\cdot2}}{x^{11}}$$
$$= \frac{36x^8}{x^{11}}$$
$$= 36x^{8-11}$$
$$= 36x^{-3}$$
$$= \frac{36}{x^3}$$

2c. Simplify: $\dfrac{y^{-3}}{(y^4)^2}$

Copyright © 2017 Pearson Education, Inc.

2d. Simplify: $\left(\dfrac{x^8}{x^4}\right)^{-5}$

$$\left(\frac{x^8}{x^4}\right)^{-5} = \left(x^4\right)^{-5}$$

$$= x^{-20}$$

$$= \frac{1}{x^{20}}$$

2d. Simplify: $\left(\dfrac{x^4}{x^2}\right)^{-3}$

Learning Objective #3: Convert from scientific notation to decimal notation.

✔ Solved Problem #3

3a. Write 7.4×10^9 in decimal notation.

The exponent is positive so we move the decimal point nine places to the right.

$$7.4 \times 10^9 = 7,400,000,000$$

3b. Write 3.017×10^{-6} in decimal notation.

The exponent is negative so we move the decimal point six places to the left.

$$3.017 \times 10^{-6} = 0.000003017$$

✎ Pencil Problem #3 ✎

3a. Write 9.23×10^5 in decimal notation.

3b. Write 7.86×10^{-4} in decimal notation.

Learning Objective #4: Convert from decimal notation to scientific notation.

✔ Solved Problem #4

4a. Write $7,410,000,000$ in scientific notation.

$$7,410,000,000 = 7.41 \times 10^9$$

✎ Pencil Problem #4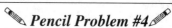

4a. Write $220,000,000$ in scientific notation.

Copyright © 2017 Pearson Education, Inc.

4b. Write 0.000000092 in scientific notation.

$$0.000000092 = 9.2 \times 10^{-8}$$

4b. Write 0.0000202 in scientific notation.

Learning Objective #5: Compute with scientific notation.

✔ Solved Problem #5

5a. Perform the indicated computation, writing the answer in scientific notation: $(3 \times 10^8)(2 \times 10^2)$

$$(3 \times 10^8)(2 \times 10^2) = (3 \times 2) \times (10^8 \times 10^2)$$
$$= 6 \times 10^{8+2}$$
$$= 6 \times 10^{10}$$

✎ Pencil Problem #5 ✎

5a. Perform the indicated computation, writing the answer in scientific notation: $(2 \times 10^3)(3 \times 10^2)$

5b. Perform the indicated computation, writing the answer in scientific notation: $\dfrac{8.4 \times 10^7}{4 \times 10^{-4}}$

$$\frac{8.4 \times 10^7}{4 \times 10^{-4}} = \frac{8.4}{4} \cdot \frac{10^7}{10^{-4}}$$
$$= 2.1 \times 10^{7-(-4)}$$
$$= 2.1 \times 10^{11}$$

5b. Perform the indicated computation, writing the answer in scientific notation: $\dfrac{15 \times 10^{-4}}{5 \times 10^2}$

5c. Perform the indicated computation, writing the answer in scientific notation: $(4 \times 10^{-2})^3$

$$(4 \times 10^{-2})^3 = 4^3 \times (10^{-2})^3$$
$$= 64 \times 10^{-6}$$
$$= 6.4 \times 10^{-5}$$

5c. Perform the indicated computation, writing the answer in scientific notation: $(3 \times 10^{-2})^4$

Copyright © 2017 Pearson Education, Inc.

Learning Objective #6: Solve applied problems using scientific notation.

✔ **Solved Problem #6**	✏ **Pencil Problem #6** ✏
6. As of December 2011, the United States had spent $2.6 trillion for the wars in Iraq and Afghanistan. (Source: costofwar.org) At that time, the U.S. population was approximately 312 million (3.12×10^8). If this cost of these wars was evenly divided among every individual in the United States, how much would each citizen have to pay?	6. If there are approximately 3.2×10^7 seconds in a year, approximately how many years is 1.09 trillion seconds?

$$\frac{2.6 \times 10^{12}}{3.12 \times 10^8} = \frac{2.6}{3.12} \times \frac{10^{12}}{10^8} \approx 0.83 \times 10^4 = 8300$$

Each citizen would have to pay about $8300.

Answers for Pencil Problems *(Textbook Exercise references in parentheses)*:

1a. $\dfrac{1}{8^2} = \dfrac{1}{64}$ *(5.7 #1)* **1b.** $\dfrac{1}{(-6)^2} = \dfrac{1}{36}$ *(5.7 #5)* **1c.** $-\dfrac{1}{6^2} = -\dfrac{1}{36}$ *(5.7 #7)*

1d. 16 *(5.7 #19)* **1e.** $\dfrac{x^5}{6}$ *(5.7 #23)* **1f.** $\dfrac{y}{x^8}$ *(5.7 # 25)*

2a. $\dfrac{1}{x^5}$ *(5.7 #29)* **2b.** $\dfrac{3}{z^5}$ *(5.7 # 37)* **2c.** $\dfrac{1}{y^{11}}$ *(5.7 # 47)* **2d.** $\dfrac{1}{x^6}$ *(5.7 #53)*

3a. 923,000 *(5.7 #81)* **3b.** 0.000786 *(5.7 #89)*

4a. 2.2×10^8 *(5.7 #93)* **4b.** 2.02×10^{-5} *(5.7 #101)*

5a. 6×10^5 *(5.7 #107)* **5b.** 3×10^{-6} *(5.7 #115)* **5c.** 8.1×10^{-7} *(5.7 #123)*

6. 34,000 years *(5.7 #141)*

Homework:

☐ **Review the Section 5.7 summary** on page 414 of the textbook.

☐ **Insert your homework** into this section of the *Learning Guide*. Show all work neatly and check your answers. Strive to work through difficulties when possible, making note of any exercises where you need additional help. Remember, even if your instructor assigns homework through *MyMathLab*, you should still write out your work.

 Copyright © 2017 Pearson Education, Inc.

Group Project for Chapter 5

A large number can be put into perspective by comparing it with another number.

Examples from the textbook:

In Example 10 on page 406 of the textbook we put the $15.2 trillion national debt into perspective by comparing this number to the number of U.S. citizens.

In Exercises 139–142 on page 410 of the textbook , we put the $1.09 trillion budget deficit into perspective by comparing 1.09 trillion to the number of U.S. citizens, the distance around the world, the number of seconds in a year, and the height of the Washington Monument.

For this project, each group member should consult an almanac, a newspaper, or the Internet to find a number greater than one million. Explain to other members of the group the context in which the large number is used. Express the number in scientific notation. Then put the number into perspective by comparing it with another number.

Copyright © 2017 Pearson Education, Inc.

Getting Ready for the Chapter 5 Test

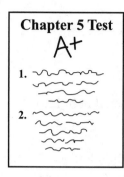

Chapter 5 Test

One of the best ways to prepare for a test is to stay on top of your studying, keeping up as your professor proceeds from section to section. Falling behind on one section often makes it difficult to understand the material in the following section. Never wait until the last minute to study for an exam.

Below are several actions that will help you stay organized as you prepare for your test.

How to prepare for your Chapter Test:

☐ **Write down any details that your instructor shares about the test.**
In addition to items such as location, date, time, and essentials to bring, be sure to listen carefully for specific information about the topics covered. Communicate with your instructor concerning any details that may be unclear to you.

☐ **Read the Chapter Summary that begins on page 411 of your textbook.**
Study the appropriate sections in the Chapter Summary. This summary contains the most important material in each section including, definitions, concepts, procedures, and examples.

☐ **Review your *Learning Guide.***
Go back through the *Solved Problems* and *Pencil Problems* in this chapter of your *Learning Guide.* You may find it helpful to cover up solutions and work through the problems again.

☐ **Study your notes and homework.**
Read through your class notes that you took during this unit, and review the corresponding homework assignments.

☐ **Review quizzes and other feedback from your professor.**
Review any quizzes you have taken and be sure you understand any errors that you made. Seek help with any concepts that are still unclear.

☐ **Complete the Review Exercises that begin on page 414 of your textbook.**
Work the assigned problems from the Review Exercises. These exercises represent the most significant problems for each of the chapter's sections. The answers for all Review Exercises are in the back of your textbook.

☐ **Take the Chapter Test that begins on page 416 of your textbook.**
- Find a quiet place to take the Chapter Test.
- Do not use notes, index cards, or any resources other than those your instructor will allow during the actual test.
- After completing the entire test, check your answers in the back of the textbook.
- Watch the *Chapter Test Prep Video* to review any exercises you may have missed.

Copyright © 2017 Pearson Education, Inc.

Chapter 6.R Factoring Polynomials
Integrated Review

Learning Objectives
1. Write the prime factorization of a number.
2. Multiply a monomial and a polynomial.
3. Use FOIL in polynomial multiplication.

Learning Objective #1: Write the prime factorization of a number.

✔ *Solved Problem #1*	*Pencil Problem #1*
1a. Find the prime factorization of 120.	**1a.** Find the prime factorization of 75.

$120 = 2^3 \cdot 3 \cdot 5$

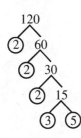

1b. Find the prime factorization of 300.

$300 = 2^2 \cdot 3 \cdot 5^2$

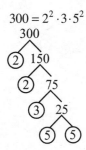

1b. Find the prime factorization of 56.

Learning Objective #2: Multiply a monomial and a polynomial.	
✔ *Solved Problem #2*	✏ *Pencil Problem #2*✏

2a. Multiply: $6x^2(5x^3 - 2x + 3)$

$$6x^2(5x^3 - 2x + 3) = 6x^2 \cdot 5x^3 - 6x^2 \cdot 2x + 6x^2 \cdot 3$$
$$= 30x^5 - 12x^3 + 18x^2$$

2a. Multiply: $-3x^2(-4x^2 + x - 5)$

2b. Multiply: $-x(2x^2 + 4x - 1)$

$$-x(2x^2 + 4x - 1) = -x \cdot 2x^2 - x \cdot 4x - x \cdot -1$$
$$= -2x^3 - 4x^2 + x$$

2b. Multiply: $2x^2(2x^2 - 3x + 2)$

Answers for Pencil Problems:

1a. $75 = 3 \cdot 5^2$ **1b.** $56 = 2^3 \cdot 7$ **2a.** $12x^4 - 3x^3 + 15x^2$ **2b.** $4x^4 - 6x^3 + 4x^2$ **3a.** $y^2 - 4y - 21$

3b. $10x^2 - 9x - 9$

Copyright © 2017 Pearson Education, Inc.

Learning Objective #3: Use FOIL in polynomial multiplication.

✔ *Solved Problem #3*	✎ *Pencil Problem #3*✎
3a. Multiply: $(x+5)(x+6)$	**3a.** Multiply: $(y-7)(y+3)$

$$(x+5)(x+6) = \overbrace{x \cdot x}^{F} + \overbrace{6 \cdot x}^{O} + \overbrace{5 \cdot x}^{I} + \overbrace{5 \cdot 6}^{L}$$
$$= x^2 + 6x + 5x + 30$$
$$= x^2 + 11x + 30$$

3b. Multiply: $(7x+5)(4x-3)$	**3b.** Multiply: $(2x-3)(5x+3)$

$$(7x+5)(4x-3) = \overbrace{7x \cdot 4x}^{F} + \overbrace{7x(-3)}^{O} + \overbrace{5 \cdot 4x}^{I} + \overbrace{5(-3)}^{L}$$
$$= 28x^2 - 21x + 20x - 15$$
$$= 28x^2 - x - 15$$

Answers for Pencil Problems:

1a. $75 = 3 \cdot 5^2$ **1b.** $56 = 2^3 \cdot 7$ **2a.** $12x^4 - 3x^3 + 15x^2$ **2b.** $4x^4 - 6x^3 + 4x^2$ **3a.** $y^2 - 4y - 21$
3b. $10x^2 - 9x - 9$

Copyright © 2017 Pearson Education, Inc.

Section 6.1
The Greatest Common Factor and Factoring by Grouping

> # *KABOOM!!!!*
>
> An explosion caused debris to rise vertically with an initial velocity of 64 feet per second. It is possible to calculate the height of the debris at any given time after the explosion.
>
> In this section of the textbook, we will look at how a polynomial can be used to model this situation, and we will apply the concept of factoring to such polynomials.

First Steps:

☐ **Take comprehensive notes** from your instructor's lecture and insert your notes into this section of the *Learning Guide*. Be sure to write down all examples, definitions, and other key concepts. Additional learning resources include the *Video Lecture Series*, the *PowerPoints*, and Section 6.1 of your textbook which begins on page 420.

☐ Complete the *Concept and Vocabulary Check* on page 426 of the textbook.

Guided Practice:

☐ Review each of the following *Solved Problems* and complete each *Pencil Problem*.

Learning Objective #1: Find the greatest common factor.	
✔ *Solved Problem #1*	✎ *Pencil Problem #1* ✎
1a. Find the greatest common factor of the following list of monomials: $18x^3$ and $15x^2$	**1a.** Find the greatest common factor of the following list of monomials: $12x^2$ and $8x$
$18x^3 = 3x^2 \cdot 6x$ $15x^2 = 3x^2 \cdot 5$ The GCF is $3x^2$.	
1b. Find the greatest common factor of the following list of monomials: x^4y, x^3y^2, and x^2y	**1b.** Find the greatest common factor of the following list of monomials: $16x^5y^4$, $8x^6y^3$, and $20x^4y^5$
$x^4y = x^2y \cdot x^2$ $x^3y^2 = x^2y \cdot xy$ $x^2y = x^2y$ The GCF is x^2y.	

Learning Objective #2: Factor out the greatest common factor of a polynomial.	
✔ *Solved Problem #2*	✎ *Pencil Problem #2*✎

2a. Factor: $6x^2 + 18$

The GCF is 6.

$6x^2 + 18 = 6 \cdot x^2 + 6 \cdot 3$
$\quad\quad\quad\quad = 6(x^2 + 3)$

2a. Factor: $18y^2 + 12$

2b. Factor: $25x^2 + 35x^3$

The GCF is $5x^2$.

$25x^2 + 35x^3 = 5x^2 \cdot 5 + 5x^2 \cdot 7x$
$\quad\quad\quad\quad\quad = 5x^2(5 + 7x)$

2b. Factor: $8x^2 - 4x^4$

2c. Factor: $15x^5 + 12x^4 - 27x^3$

The GCF is $3x^3$.

$15x^5 + 12x^4 - 27x^3 = 3x^3 \cdot 5x^2 + 3x^3 \cdot 4x - 3x^3 \cdot 9$
$\quad\quad\quad\quad\quad\quad\quad\quad = 3x^3(5x^2 + 4x - 9)$

2c. Factor: $100y^5 - 50y^3 + 100y^2$

2d. Factor: $8x^3y^2 - 14x^2y + 2xy$

The GCF is $2xy$.

$8x^3y^2 - 14x^2y + 2xy = 2xy \cdot 4x^2y - 2xy \cdot 7x + 2xy \cdot 1$
$\quad\quad\quad\quad\quad\quad\quad\quad = 2xy(4x^2y - 7x + 1)$

2d. Factor: $11x^2 - 23$

Copyright © 2017 Pearson Education, Inc.

Learning Objective #3: Factor out the negative of the greatest common factor of a polynomial.

✔ **Solved Problem #3**	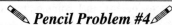 **Pencil Problem #3**

3. Factor: $-16a^4b^5 + 24a^3b^4 - 20ab^2$

3. Factor: $-4a^3b^2 + 6ab$

It is preferable to have a first term with a positive coefficient inside parentheses.

Thus, we will factor out $-4ab^2$.

$-16a^4b^5 + 24a^3b^4 - 20ab^2$

$= -4ab^2 \cdot 4a^3b^3 - 4ab^2 \cdot (-6a^2b^2) - 4ab^2 \cdot 5$

$= -4ab^2(4a^3b^3 - 6a^2b^2 + 5)$

Learning Objective #4: Factor by grouping.

✔ **Solved Problem #4**	✎ **Pencil Problem #4**

4a. Factor: $x^2(x+1) + 7(x+1)$

4a. Factor: $x(x+5) + 3(x+5)$

Factor out the greatest common factor of $x+1$.

$$x^2 \overbrace{(x+1)}^{\text{GCF}} + 7 \overbrace{(x+1)}^{\text{GCF}} = (x+1)(x^2+7)$$

4b. Factor: $x(y+4) - 7(y+4)$

4b. Factor: $3x(x+y) - (x+y)$

Factor out the greatest common factor of $y+4$.

$$x \overbrace{(y+4)}^{\text{GCF}} - 7 \overbrace{(y+4)}^{\text{GCF}} = (y+4)(x-7)$$

4c. Factor: $x^3 + 5x^2 + 2x + 10$

There is no factor other than 1 common to all four terms. However, we can group terms that have a common factor.

$$x^3 + 5x^2 + 2x + 10 = (x^3 + 5x^2) + (2x + 10)$$

Factor out the greatest common factor from the grouped terms. The remaining two terms have $x + 5$ as a common binomial factor, which should then be factored out.

$$x^3 + 5x^2 + 2x + 10 = (x^3 + 5x^2) + (2x + 10)$$
$$= x^2(x + 5) + 2(x + 5)$$
$$= (x + 5)(x^2 + 2)$$

4c. Factor: $x^2 + 2x + 4x + 8$

4d. Factor: $xy + 3x - 5y - 15$

There is no factor other than 1 common to all four terms. However, we can group terms that have a common factor.

$$xy + 3x - 5y - 15 = (xy + 3x) + (-5y - 15)$$

Factor out x from the first two grouped terms and -5 from the last two grouped terms.

$$xy + 3x - 5y - 15 = x(y + 3) - 5(y + 3)$$

Finally, factor out the common factor of $y + 3$.

$$xy + 3x - 5y - 15 = x(y + 3) - 5(y + 3)$$
$$= (y + 3)(x - 5)$$

4d. Factor: $3x^3 - 2x^2 - 6x + 4$

Answers for Pencil Problems *(Textbook Exercise references in parentheses)*:

1a. $4x$ *(6.1 #3)*   **1b.** $4x^4 y^3$ *(6.1 #11)*   **2a.** $6(3y^2 + 2)$ *(6.1 #23)*   **2b.** $4x^2(2 - x^2)$ *(6.1 #31)*

2c. $50y^2(2y^3 - y + 2)$ *(6.1 #37)*   **2d.** cannot be factored *(6.1 #41)*   **3.** $-2ab(2a^2 b - 3)$ *(6.1 #53)*

4a. $(x + 5)(x + 3)$ *(6.1 #57)*   **4b.** $(x + y)(3x - 1)$ *(6.1 #63)*

4c. $(x + 2)(x + 4)$ *(6.1 #69)*   **4d.** $(3x - 2)(x^2 - 2)$ *(6.1 #83)*

Homework:

☐ **Review the Section 6.1 summary** on page 477 of the textbook.

☐ **Insert your homework** into this section of the *Learning Guide*. Show all work neatly and check your answers. Strive to work through difficulties when possible, making note of any exercises where you need additional help. Remember, even if your instructor assigns homework through *MyMathLab*, you should still write out your work.

Copyright © 2017 Pearson Education, Inc.

Section 6.2
Factoring Trinomials Whose Leading Coefficient is 1

Dive In!

Did you know that when you jump upward from a diving board, your height at any given time can be calculated using a trinomial expression?

An application exercise in this section of the textbook will explore this situation in detail.

First Steps:

☐ **Take comprehensive notes** from your instructor's lecture and insert your notes into this section of the *Learning Guide*. Be sure to write down all examples, definitions, and other key concepts. Additional learning resources include the *Video Lecture Series*, the *PowerPoints*, and Section 6.2 of your textbook which begins on page 429.

☐ Complete the *Concept and Vocabulary Check* on page 435 of the textbook.

Guided Practice:

☐ Review each of the following *Solved Problems* and complete each *Pencil Problem*.

Learning Objective #1: Factor trinomials of the form $x^2 + bx + c$.

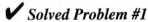 **Solved Problem #1**   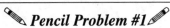 *Pencil Problem #1*

1a. Factor: $x^2 + 5x + 6$ **1a.** Factor: $x^2 + 7x + 10$

Factors of 6	6,1	−6,−1	2,3	−2,−3
Sum of Factors	7	−7	5	−5

The factors of 6 whose sum is 5, are 2 and 3.

Thus, $x^2 + 5x + 6 = (x+2)(x+3)$.

Check:
$$(x+2)(x+3) = x^2 + 3x + 2x + 6$$
$$= x^2 + 5x + 6$$

1b. Factor: $x^2 - 6x + 8$

Factors of 8	8,1	−8,−1	2,4	−2,−4
Sum of Factors	9	−9	6	−6

The factors of 8 whose sum is −6, are −2 and −4.

Thus, $x^2 - 6x + 8 = (x - 2)(x - 4)$.

Check:

$(x - 2)(x - 4) = x^2 - 4x - 2x + 8$
$= x^2 - 6x + 8$

1b. Factor: $x^2 - 7x + 12$

1c. Factor: $x^2 + 3x - 10$

Factors of −10	−10,1	10,−1	−5,2	5,−2
Sum of Factors	−9	9	−3	3

The factors of −10 whose sum is 3, are 5 and −2.

Thus, $x^2 + 3x - 10 = (x + 5)(x - 2)$.

Check:

$(x + 5)(x - 2) = x^2 - 2x + 5x - 10$
$= x^2 + 3x - 10$

1c. Factor: $y^2 + 10y - 39$

1d. Factor: $y^2 - 6y - 27$

The factors of −27 whose sum is −6, are −9 and 3.

Thus, $y^2 - 6y - 27 = (y - 9)(y + 3)$.

1d. Factor: $x^2 - 2x - 15$

Copyright © 2017 Pearson Education, Inc.

1e. Factor: $x^2 + x - 7$

No factor pair of –7 has a sum of 1.

Thus, $x^2 + x - 7$ is prime.

1e. Factor: $x^2 + 4x + 12$

1f. Factor: $x^2 - 4xy + 3y^2$

The factors of 3 whose sum is –4, are –3 and –1.

Thus, $x^2 - 4xy + 3y^2 = (x - 3y)(x - y)$.

1f. Factor: $x^2 + 7xy + 6y^2$

1g. Factor: $2x^3 + 6x^2 - 56x$

First factor out the common factor of $2x$.
$2x^3 + 6x^2 - 56x = 2x(x^2 + 3x - 28)$

Continue by factoring the trinomial.
$$2x^3 + 6x^2 - 56x = 2x(x^2 + 3x - 28)$$
$$= 2x(x - 4)(x + 7)$$

1g. Factor: $3x^2 + 15x + 18$

Copyright © 2017 Pearson Education, Inc.

1h. Factor: $-2y^2 - 10y + 28$

1h. Factor: $-2x^3 - 6x^2 + 8x$

First factor out the common factor of -2.
$$-2y^2 - 10y + 28 = -2(y^2 + 5y - 14)$$

Continue by factoring the trinomial.
$$-2y^2 - 10y + 28 = -2(y^2 + 5y - 14)$$
$$= -2(y - 2)(y + 7)$$

Answers for Pencil Problems *(Textbook Exercise references in parentheses)*:

1a. $(x + 5)(x + 2)$ *(6.2 #3)*

1b. $(x - 4)(x - 3)$ *(6.2 #7)*

1c. $(y + 13)(y - 3)$ *(6.2 #15)*

1d. $(x - 5)(x + 3)$ *(6.2 #17)*

1e. prime   *(6.2 #21)*

1f. $(x + 6y)(x + y)$ *(6.2 #35)*

1g. $3(x + 2)(x + 3)$ *(6.2 #43)*

1h. $-2x(x + 4)(x - 1)$ *(6.2 #73)*

Homework:

☐ **Review the Section 6.2 summary** on page 477 of the textbook.

☐ **Insert your homework** into this section of the *Learning Guide*. Show all work neatly and check your answers. Strive to work through difficulties when possible, making note of any exercises where you need additional help. Remember, even if your instructor assigns homework through *MyMathLab*, you should still write out your work.

Copyright © 2017 Pearson Education, Inc.

Section 6.3
Factoring Trinomials Whose Leading Coefficient Is Not 1

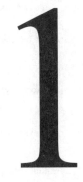

Is ONE the Loneliest Number?

The number 1 does not appear to be lonely when it comes to language.

The words
"unit," "unity," "union," "unique," and "universal"
are all derived from the Latin word for "one."

For the ancient Greeks, 1 was the indivisible unit from which
all other numbers arose.

The Greek's philosophy of 1 applies to our work in this section.
Factoring trinomials whose leading coefficient is 1 is the basic
technique from which other methods of factoring will follow.

In this section of the text, we factor trinomials with leading coefficients that are not 1.

First Steps:

☐ **Take comprehensive notes** from your instructor's lecture and insert your notes into this section of the *Learning Guide*. Be sure to write down all examples, definitions, and other key concepts. Additional learning resources include the *Video Lecture Series*, the *PowerPoints*, and Section 6.3 of your textbook which begins on page 438.

☐ Complete the *Concept and Vocabulary Check* on page 443 of the textbook.

Here is an observation that sometimes helps narrow down the list of possible factorizations.

If a polynomial does not have a GCF other than 1 or if you have factored out the GCF, there will be no common factor within any of its binomial factors.

Here is an example:

$$6x^2 - 17x + 12$$ ← There is no GCF other than 1.

$$(2x - 4)(3x + 3)$$ ← This is not a possible factorization.

This binomial has a common factor of 2.

This binomial has a common factor of 3.

Copyright © 2017 Pearson Education, Inc.

Guided Practice:

☐ Review each of the following *Solved Problems* and complete each *Pencil Problem*.

Learning Objective #1: Factor trinomials by trial and error.

✔ Solved Problem #1

1a. Factor $6x^2 + 19x - 7$ by trial and error.

Step 1 Find two first terms whose product is $6x^2$.

$$6x^2 + 19x - 7 = (6x \quad)(x \quad)$$
$$6x^2 + 19x - 7 = (3x \quad)(2x \quad)$$

Step 2 The last term, -7, has possible factorizations of $1(-7)$ and $-1(7)$.

Step 3

Possible Factors of $6x^2 + 19x - 7$	Sum of Outside and Inside Products
$(6x+1)(x-7)$	$-42x + x = -41x$
$(6x-7)(x+1)$	$6x - 7x = -x$
$(6x-1)(x+7)$	$42x - x = 41x$
$(6x+7)(x-1)$	$-6x + 7x = x$
$(3x+1)(2x-7)$	$-21x + 2x = -19x$
$(3x-7)(2x+1)$	$3x - 14x = -11x$
$(3x-1)(2x+7)$	required middle term $21x - 2x = 19x$
$(3x+7)(2x-1)$	$-3x + 14x = 11x$

The required middle term is obtained by using the factors $(3x-1)(2x+7)$.

Check: $(3x-1)(2x+7) = 6x^2 + 21x - 2x - 7$
$$= 6x^2 + 19x - 7$$

Thus, $6x^2 + 19x - 7 = (3x-1)(2x+7)$

✎ Pencil Problem #1 ✎

1a. Factor $2x^2 + 5x + 3$ by trial and error.

Copyright © 2017 Pearson Education, Inc.

1b. Factor $3x^2 - 13xy + 4y^2$ by trial and error.

Step 1 Find two First terms whose product is $3x^2$.

$$3x^2 - 13xy + 4y^2 = (3x \quad)(x \quad)$$

Step 2 The last term, $4y^2$, has pairs of factors that are either both positive or both negative. Because the middle term, $-13xy$, is negative, both factors must be negative. Thus the last term has possible factorizations of $-2y(-2y)$ or $-y(-4y)$.

Step 3

Possible Factors of $3x^2 - 13xy + 4y^2$	Sum of Outside and Inside Products
$(3x - 4y)(x - y)$	$-3xy - 4xy = -7xy$
$(3x - y)(x - 4y)$	required middle term $-12xy - xy = -13xy$
$(3x - 2y)(x - 2y)$	$-6xy - 2xy = -8xy$

The required middle term is obtained by using the factors $(3x - y)(x - 4y)$.

Check: $(3x - y)(x - 4y) = 3x^2 - 12xy - xy + 4y^2$
$$= 3x^2 - 13xy + 4y^2$$

Thus, $3x^2 - 13xy + 4y^2 = (3x - y)(x - 4y)$

1b. Factor $3x^2 + 5xy + 2y^2$ by trial and error.

Learning Objective #2: Factor trinomials by grouping.

✔ Solved Problem #2

2a. Factor $3x^2 - x - 10$ by grouping.

$a = 3$ and $c = -10$, so $ac = 3(-10) = -30$.

The factors of -30 whose sum is -1 are 5 and -6.

$3x^2 - x - 10 = 3x^2 + 5x - 6x - 10$
$$= x(3x + 5) - 2(3x + 5)$$
$$= (3x + 5)(x - 2)$$

Check: $(3x + 5)(x - 2) = 3x^2 - 6x + 5x - 10$
$$= 3x^2 - x - 10$$

Thus, $3x^2 - x - 10 = (3x + 5)(x - 2)$

✎ Pencil Problem #2 ✎

2a. Factor $9y^2 - 9y + 2$ by grouping.

2b. Factor $8x^2 - 10x + 3$ by grouping.

$a = 8$ and $c = 3$, so $ac = 8(3) = 24$.

The factors of 24 whose sum is -10 are -6 and -4.

$$8x^2 - 10x + 3 = 8x^2 - 4x - 6x + 3$$
$$= 4x(2x - 1) - 3(2x - 1)$$
$$= (2x - 1)(4x - 3)$$

2b. Factor $20x^2 + 27x - 8$ by grouping.

2c. Factor completely: $5y^4 + 13y^3 + 6y^2$

First factor out the greatest common factor (GCF) of y^2.
$$5y^4 + 13y^3 + 6y^2 = y^2(5y^2 + 13y + 6)$$

Then factor the resulting trinomial.
$$5y^4 + 13y^3 + 6y^2 = y^2(5y^2 + 13y + 6)$$
$$= y^2(5y + 3)(y + 2)$$

2c. Factor completely: $4x^2 + 26x + 30$

Answers for Pencil Problems *(Textbook Exercise references in parentheses)*:

1a. $(2x + 3)(x + 1)$ *(6.3 #1)*   **1b.** $(3x + 2y)(x + y)$ *(6.3 #45)*

2a. $(3y - 1)(3y - 2)$ *(6.3 #39)*   **2b.** $(4x - 1)(5x + 8)$ *(6.3 #41)*   **2c.** $2(2x + 3)(x + 5)$ *(6.3 #59)*

Homework:

☐ **Review the Section 6.3 summary** on page 477 of the textbook.

☐ **Insert your homework** into this section of the *Learning Guide*. Show all work neatly and check your answers. Strive to work through difficulties when possible, making note of any exercises where you need additional help. Remember, even if your instructor assigns homework through *MyMathLab*, you should still write out your work.

   Copyright © 2017 Pearson Education, Inc.

Section 6.4
Factoring Special Forms

Do you enjoy Solving P_z_l_s?

The process of solving puzzles is a natural way to develop problem-solving skills that are important to every area of our lives. Engaging in problem solving for sheer pleasure releases chemicals in the brain that enhance our feeling of well-being. Perhaps this is why puzzles date back 12,000 years.

In this section, we develop factoring techniques by reversing the formulas for special products discussed in the previous chapter. These factorizations can be visualized by fitting pieces of a puzzle together to form rectangles.

First Steps:

☐ **Take comprehensive notes** from your instructor's lecture and insert your notes into this section of the *Learning Guide*. Be sure to write down all examples, definitions, and other key concepts. Additional learning resources include the *Video Lecture Series*, the *PowerPoints*, and Section 6.4 of your textbook which begins on page 446.

☐ Complete the *Concept and Vocabulary Check* on page 453 of the textbook.

Guided Practice:

☐ Review each of the following *Solved Problems* and complete each *Pencil Problem*.

Learning Objective #1: Factor the difference of two squares.

✔ *Solved Problem #1*	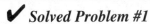 *Pencil Problem #1*
1a. Factor: $x^2 - 81$	**1a.** Factor: $x^2 - 25$

Notice that the trinomial fits the form $A^2 - B^2$.

Thus, factor using $A^2 - B^2 = (A + B)(A - B)$.

$$x^2 - 81 = x^2 - 9^2$$
$$= (x + 9)(x - 9)$$

1b. Factor: $36x^2 - 25$

Notice that the trinomial fits the form $A^2 - B^2$.

Thus, factor using $A^2 - B^2 = (A+B)(A-B)$.

$36x^2 - 25 = (6x)^2 - 5^2$
$\qquad\quad = (6x+5)(6x-5)$

1b. Factor: $x^2 + 36$

1c. Factor: $25 - 4x^{10}$

Notice that the trinomial fits the form $A^2 - B^2$.

Thus, factor using $A^2 - B^2 = (A+B)(A-B)$.

$25 - 4x^{10} = 5^2 - (2x^5)^2$
$\qquad\qquad = (5+2x^5)(5-2x^5)$

1c. Factor: $49y^4 - 16$

1d. Factor: $18x^3 - 2x$

First factor out the GCF.
$18x^3 - 2x = 2x(9x^2 - 1)$

Next, factor the difference of two squares.
$18x^3 - 2x = 2x(9x^2 - 1)$
$\qquad\qquad = 2x(3x+1)(3x-1)$

1d. Factor: $2x^3 - 72x$

1e. Factor: $81x^4 - 16$

First, factor the difference of two squares.
$81x^4 - 16 = (9x^2 + 4)(9x^2 - 4)$

The factor of $9x^2 - 4$ is the difference of two squares and can be factored.

$81x^4 - 16 = (9x^2 + 4)(9x^2 - 4)$
$\qquad\qquad = (9x^2 + 4)(3x+2)(3x-2)$

1e. Factor: $x^4 - 16$

Copyright © 2017 Pearson Education, Inc.

Learning Objective #2: Factor perfect square trinomials.

✔ Solved Problem #2

2a. Factor: $x^2 + 14x + 49$

Notice that the trinomial fits the form $A^2 + 2AB + B^2$.

Thus, factor using $A^2 + 2AB + B^2 = (A + B)^2$.

$x^2 + 14x + 49 = (x + 7)^2$

2b. Factor: $16x^2 - 56x + 49$

Notice that the trinomial fits the form $A^2 - 2AB + B^2$.

Thus, factor using $A^2 - 2AB + B^2 = (A - B)^2$.

$16x^2 - 56x + 49 = (4x - 7)^2$

2c. Factor: $4x^2 + 12xy + 9y^2$

Notice that the trinomial fits the form $A^2 + 2AB + B^2$.

Thus, factor using $A^2 + 2AB + B^2 = (A + B)^2$.

$4x^2 + 12xy + 9y^2 = (2x + 3y)^2$

✏ Pencil Problem #2 ✏

2a. Factor: $x^2 + 2x + 1$

2b. Factor: $25y^2 - 10y + 1$

2c. Factor: $16x^2 - 40xy + 25y^2$

Learning Objective #3: Factor the sum or difference of two cubes.

✔ Solved Problem #3

3a. Factor: $x^3 + 27$

Notice that the polynomial fits the form $A^3 + B^3$.

Thus it factors as $(A + B)(A^2 - AB + B^2)$.

$x^3 + 27 = x^3 + 3^3$
$\qquad = (x + 3)(x^2 - 3x + 3^2)$
$\qquad = (x + 3)(x^2 - 3x + 9)$

✏ Pencil Problem #3 ✏

3a. Factor: $x^3 + 1$

3b. Factor: $1 - y^3$

Notice that the polynomial fits the form $A^3 - B^3$.

Thus it factors as $(A - B)(A^2 + AB + B^2)$.

$1 - y^3 = 1^3 - y^3$
$\quad\quad = (1 - y)(1^2 + 1 \cdot y + y^2)$
$\quad\quad = (1 - y)(1 + y + y^2)$

3b. Factor: $8y^3 - 1$

3c. Factor: $125x^3 + 8$

Notice that the polynomial fits the form $A^3 + B^3$.

Thus it factors as $(A + B)(A^2 - AB + B^2)$.

$125x^3 + 8 = (5x)^3 + 2^3$
$\quad\quad = (5x + 2)\left[(5x)^2 - (5x)(2) + 2^2\right]$
$\quad\quad = (5x + 2)(25x^2 - 10x + 4)$

3c. Factor: $64x^3 + 27y^3$

Answers for Pencil Problems *(Textbook Exercise references in parentheses)*:

1a. $(x + 5)(x - 5)$ *(6.4 #1)*   **1b.** prime *(6.4 #31)*   **1c.** $(7y^2 + 4)(7y^2 - 4)$ *(6.4 #15)*

1d. $2x(x + 6)(x - 6)$ *(6.4 #29)*   **1e.** $(x^2 + 4)(x + 2)(x - 2)$ *(6.4 #23)*   **2a.** $(x + 1)^2$ *(6.4 #45)*

2b. $(5y - 1)^2$ *(6.4 #55)*   **2c.** $(4x - 5y)^2$ *(6.4 #65)*   **3a.** $(x + 1)(x^2 - x + 1)$ *(6.4 #79)*

3b. $(2y - 1)(4y^2 + 2y + 1)$ *(6.4 #83)*   **3c.** $(4x + 3y)(16x^2 - 12xy + 9y^2)$ *(6.4 #93)*

Homework:

☐ **Review the Section 6.4 summary** on page 478 of the textbook.

☐ **Insert your homework** into this section of the *Learning Guide*. Show all work neatly and check your answers. Strive to work through difficulties when possible, making note of any exercises where you need additional help. Remember, even if your instructor assigns homework through *MyMathLab*, you should still write out your work.

    Copyright © 2017 Pearson Education, Inc.

Section 6.5
A General Factoring Strategy

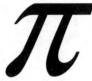

As Easy as Pi !

The number pi, symbolized as π, is a special number that denotes the ratio of a circle's circumference to its diameter. Pi is necessary when calculating the area of a circle.

In the Exercise Set for this section of the textbook, we will use π, and factoring, to write an expression that represents the area of a circular ring.

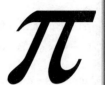

First Steps:

☐ **Take comprehensive notes** from your instructor's lecture and insert your notes into this section of the *Learning Guide*. Be sure to write down all examples, definitions, and other key concepts. Additional learning resources include the *Video Lecture Series*, the *PowerPoints*, and Section 6.5 of your textbook which begins on page 456.

☐ Complete the **Concept and Vocabulary Check** on page 461 of the textbook.

Guided Practice:

☐ Review each of the following **Solved Problems** and complete each **Pencil Problem**.

Learning Objective #1: Recognize the appropriate method for factoring a polynomial.	
✔ *Solved Problem #1*	✏ *Pencil Problem #1* ✏
1a. Name the appropriate factoring method: $$24y^2 - 36y$$ Common factoring	**1a.** Name the appropriate factoring method: $$-7x^2 + 35x$$
1b. Name the appropriate factoring method: $$w^2 - 100$$ Difference of two squares	**1b.** Name the appropriate factoring method: $$25x^2 - 49$$
1c. Name the appropriate factoring method: $$y^3 + 125$$ Sum of two cubes	**1c.** Name the appropriate factoring method: $$27x^3 - 1$$
1d. Name the appropriate factoring method: $$3xy - y + 6x - 2$$ Factor by grouping	**1d.** Name the appropriate factoring method: $$5x + 5y + x^2 + xy$$

Learning Objective #2: Use a general strategy for factoring polynomials.	
✔ *Solved Problem #2*	✏ *Pencil Problem #2* ✏

2a. Factor: $5x^4 - 45x^2$

First use common factoring.
$5x^4 - 45x^2 = 5x^2(x^2 - 9)$

Then use the difference of two squares.
$5x^4 - 45x^2 = 5x^2(x^2 - 9)$
$\qquad\qquad = 5x^2(x+3)(x-3)$

2a. Factor: $7x^3 + 7x$

2b. Factor: $4x^2 - 16x - 48$

First use common factoring.
$4x^2 - 16x - 48 = 4(x^2 - 4x - 12)$

Then use trial and error or grouping.
$4x^2 - 16x - 48 = 4(x^2 - 4x - 12)$
$\qquad\qquad\quad = 4(x-6)(x+2)$

2b. Factor: $5x^2 - 5x - 30$

2c. Factor: $4x^5 - 64x$

First use common factoring.
$4x^5 - 64x = 4x(x^4 - 16)$

Then use the difference of two squares.
$4x^5 - 64x = 4x(x^4 - 16)$
$\qquad\qquad = 4x(x^2 + 4)(x^2 - 4)$

Finally, use the difference of two squares again.
$4x^5 - 64x = 4x(x^4 - 16)$
$\qquad\qquad = 4x(x^2 + 4)(x^2 - 4)$
$\qquad\qquad = 4x(x^2 + 4)(x+2)(x-2)$

2c. Factor: $2x^4 - 162$

Copyright © 2017 Pearson Education, Inc.

2d. Factor: $x^3 - 4x^2 - 9x + 36$

Use factor by grouping.
$$x^3 - 4x^2 - 9x + 36 = x^2(x-4) - 9(x-4)$$
$$= (x-4)(x^2-9)$$

Then use the difference of two squares.
$$x^3 - 4x^2 - 9x + 36 = x^2(x-4) - 9(x-4)$$
$$= (x-4)(x^2-9)$$
$$= (x-4)(x+3)(x-3)$$

2d. Factor: $xy - 7x + 3y - 21$

2e. Factor: $3x^3 - 30x^2 + 75x$

First use common factoring.
$$3x^3 - 30x^2 + 75x = 3x(x^2 - 10x + 25)$$

The trinomial is a perfect square trinomial.
$$3x^3 - 30x^2 + 75x = 3x(x^2 - 10x + 25)$$
$$= 3x(x-5)^2$$

2e. Factor: $7y^4 + 14y^3 + 7y^2$

2f. Factor: $2x^5 + 54x^2$

First use common factoring.
$$2x^5 + 54x^2 = 2x^2(x^3 + 27)$$

The binomial is the sum of two cubes.
$$2x^5 + 54x^2 = 2x^2(x^3 + 27)$$
$$= 2x^2(x+3)(x^2 - 3x + 9)$$

2f. Factor: $2x^5 + 2x^2$

Copyright © 2017 Pearson Education, Inc.

2g. Factor: $3x^4 y - 48 y^5$

First use common factoring.
$3x^4 y - 48 y^5 = 3y(x^4 - 16 y^4)$

Then use the difference of two squares.
$$3x^4 y - 48 y^5 = 3y(x^4 - 16 y^4)$$
$$= 3y(x^2 + 4y^2)(x^2 - 4y^2)$$

Finally, use the difference of two squares again.
$$3x^4 y - 48 y^5 = 3y(x^4 - 16 y^4)$$
$$= 3y(x^2 + 4y^2)(x^2 - 4y^2)$$
$$= 3y(x^2 + 4y^2)(x + 2y)(x - 2y)$$

2g. Factor: $48x^4 y - 3x^2 y$

2h. Factor: $12x^3 + 36x^2 y + 27xy^2$

First use common factoring.
$12x^3 + 36x^2 y + 27xy^2 = 3x(4x^2 + 12xy + 9y^2)$

The trinomial is a perfect square trinomial.
$$12x^3 + 36x^2 y + 27xy^2 = 3x(4x^2 + 12xy + 9y^2)$$
$$= 3x(2x + 3y)^2$$

2h. Factor: $2bx^2 + 44bx + 242b$

Answers for Pencil Problems *(Textbook Exercise references in parentheses)*:

1a. common factoring *(6.5 #1)*   **1b.** difference of two squares *(6.5 #3)*   **1c.** difference of two cubes *(6.5 #5)*

1d. factor by grouping *(6.5 #7)*   **2a.** $7x(x^2 + 1)$ *(6.5 #19)*   **2b.** $5(x + 2)(x - 3)$ *(6.5 #21)*

2c. $2(x^2 + 9)(x + 3)(x - 3)$ *(6.5 #23)*   **2d.** $(y - 7)(x + 3)$ *(6.5 #83)*   **2e.** $7y^2(y + 1)^2$ *(6.5 #35)*

2f. $2x^2(x + 1)(x^2 - x + 1)$ *(6.5 #29)*   **2g.** $3x^2 y(4x + 1)(4x - 1)$ *(6.5 #91)*   **2h.** $2b(x + 11)^2$ *(6.5 #99)*

Homework:

☐ **Review the Section 6.5 summary** on page 478 of the textbook.

☐ **Insert your homework** into this section of the *Learning Guide*. Show all work neatly and check your answers. Strive to work through difficulties when possible, making note of any exercises where you need additional help. Remember, even if your instructor assigns homework through *MyMathLab*, you should still write out your work.

                    Copyright © 2017 Pearson Education, Inc.

Section 6.6
Solving Quadratic Equations by Factoring

See you later, Alligator?

Fortunately, the alligator is no longer an endangered species. At one time the alligator was the subject of a protection program at Florida's Everglades National Park.

Park rangers used a formula to estimate the alligator population during the years of the program.

In this section of the textbook, you will solve a quadratic equation in order to estimate the number of years it took for the alligator population to reach various levels.

First Steps:

☐ **Take comprehensive notes** from your instructor's lecture and insert your notes into this section of the *Learning Guide*. Be sure to write down all examples, definitions, and other key concepts. Additional learning resources include the *Video Lecture Series*, the *PowerPoints*, and Section 6.6 of your textbook which begins on page 464.

☐ Complete the *Concept and Vocabulary Check* on page 473 of the textbook.

Guided Practice:

☐ Review each of the following *Solved Problems* and complete each *Pencil Problem*.

Learning Objective #1: Use the zero-product principle.

✔ *Solved Problem #1*	✎ *Pencil Problem #1* ✎
1. Solve the equation: $(2x+1)(x-4)=0$	**1.** Solve the equation: $(x-6)(x+4)=0$

The equation is in factored form on the left side with zero on the right side. Thus, set each factor equal to zero and solve the resulting equations.

$$2x+1=0 \quad \text{or} \quad x-4=0$$
$$2x=-1 \qquad\qquad x=4$$
$$x=-\frac{1}{2}$$

The solution set is $\left\{-\frac{1}{2}, 4\right\}$.

Learning Objective #2: Solve quadratic equations by factoring.	

✔ *Solved Problem #2*	✎ *Pencil Problem #2* ✎

2a. Solve: $x^2 - 6x + 5 = 0$

All the terms are on one side and zero is on the other side.

$x^2 - 6x + 5 = 0$

Thus, factor the left side of the equation.

$x^2 - 6x + 5 = 0$

$(x-1)(x-5) = 0$

Next, set each factor equal to zero and solve the resulting equations.

$x - 1 = 0$ or $x - 5 = 0$

$\quad x = 1$ $\qquad\qquad x = 5$

The solution set is $\{1, 5\}$.

2a. Solve: $x^2 - 5x = 0$

2b. Solve: $4x^2 = 2x$

Move all terms to one side and obtain zero on the other side.

$4x^2 = 2x$

$4x^2 - 2x = 0$

Then factor the left side of the equation.

$4x^2 - 2x = 0$

$2x(2x - 1) = 0$

Next, set each factor equal to zero and solve the resulting equations.

$2x = 0$ or $2x - 1 = 0$

$\quad x = 0$ $\qquad\quad 2x = 1$

$\qquad\qquad\qquad x = \dfrac{1}{2}$

The solution set is $\left\{0, \dfrac{1}{2}\right\}$.

2b. Solve: $2x^2 = 7x + 4$

Copyright © 2017 Pearson Education, Inc.

2c. Solve: $x^2 = 10x - 25$

Move all terms to one side and obtain zero on the other side.

$$x^2 = 10x - 25$$
$$x^2 - 10x + 25 = 0$$

Then factor the left side of the equation.

$$x^2 - 10x + 25 = 0$$
$$(x - 5)^2 = 0$$

Because both factors are the same, it is only necessary to set one of them equal to zero.

$$x - 5 = 0$$
$$x = 5$$

The solution set is $\{5\}$.

2c. Solve: $x^2 + 4x + 4 = 0$

2d. Solve: $(x - 5)(x - 2) = 28$

Write the equation in standard form by finding the product on the left side and then subtracting 28 from both sides.

$$(x - 5)(x - 2) = 28$$
$$x^2 - 7x + 10 = 28$$
$$x^2 - 7x - 18 = 0$$

Then factor the left side of the equation.

$$x^2 - 7x - 18 = 0$$
$$(x - 9)(x + 2) = 0$$

Set each factor equal to zero and solve the resulting equations.

$$x^2 - 7x - 18 = 0$$
$$(x - 9)(x + 2) = 0$$
$$x - 9 = 0 \quad \text{or} \quad x + 2 = 0$$
$$x = 9 \qquad\qquad x = -2$$

The solution set is $\{-2, 9\}$.

2d. Solve: $x(x - 4) = 21$

Copyright © 2017 Pearson Education, Inc.

Learning Objective #3: Solve problems using quadratic equations.

✔ Solved Problem #3

3. The length of a rectangular sign is 3 feet longer than the width. If the sign's area is 54 square feet, find its length and width.

Let $x =$ the width of the sign.
Let $x + 3 =$ the length of the sign.

The area of 54 square feet can be represented as follows.
$A = l \cdot w$
$54 = (x + 3) \cdot x$

Write the equation in standard form by finding the product on the right side and then subtracting 54 from both sides.
$54 = (x + 3) \cdot x$

$54 = x^2 + 3x$

$0 = x^2 + 3x - 54$

$0 = (x - 6)(x + 9)$

Set each factor equal to zero and solve the resulting equations.
$x - 6 = 0$ or $x + 9 = 0$
    $x = 6$ $x = -9$

Reject –9 because the width cannot be negative.

The width of the sign is 6 feet and the length is $6 + 3$, or 9 feet.

✎ Pencil Problem #3 ✎

3. The number of football games, N, that must be played in a league with t teams if each team is to play every other team once is described by

$$N = \frac{t^2 - t}{2}.$$

If a league has 45 games scheduled, how many teams belong to the league, assuming that each team plays every other team once?

Answers for Pencil Problems *(Textbook Exercise references in parentheses)*:

1. $\{-4, 6\}$ *(6.6 #3)*   **2a.** $\{0, 5\}$ *(6.6 #19)*   **2b.** $\left\{-\frac{1}{2}, 4\right\}$ *(6.6 #33)*   **2c.** $\{-2\}$ *(6.6 #27)*

2d. $\{-3, 7\}$ *(6.6 #43)*   **3.** 10 teams   *(6.6 #81)*

Homework:

☐ **Review the Section 6.6 summary** on page 478 of the textbook.

☐ **Insert your homework** into this section of the *Learning Guide.* Show all work neatly and check your answers. Strive to work through difficulties when possible, making note of any exercises where you need additional help. Remember, even if your instructor assigns homework through *MyMathLab*, you should still write out your work.

 Copyright © 2017 Pearson Education, Inc.

Group members are on the board of a condominium association. The condominium has just installed a 35-foot-by-30-foot pool. Your job is to choose a material to surround the pool to create a border of uniform width.

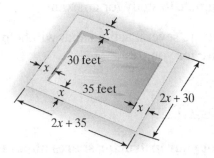

a. Begin by writing an algebraic expression for the area, in square feet, of the border around the pool. (Hint: The border's area is the combined area of the pool and border minus the area of the pool.)

b. You must select one of the following options for the border.

Options for the Border	Price
Cement	$6 per square foot
Outdoor carpeting	$5 per square foot plus $10 per foot to install edging around the rectangular border
Brick	$8 per square foot plus a $60 charge for delivering the bricks

Write an algebraic expression for the cost of installing the border for each of these options.

c. You would like the border to be 5 feet wide. Use the algebraic expressions in part (b) to find the cost of the border for each of the three options.

d. You would prefer not to use cement. However, the condominium association is limited by a $5000 budget. Given this limitation, approximately how wide can the border be using outdoor carpeting or brick? Which option should you select and why?

Copyright © 2017 Pearson Education, Inc.

Getting Ready for the Chapter 6 Test

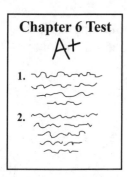

Chapter 6 Test
A+

One of the best ways to prepare for a test is to stay on top of your studying, keeping up as your professor proceeds from section to section. Falling behind on one section often makes it difficult to understand the material in the following section. Never wait until the last minute to study for an exam.

Below are several actions that will help you stay organized as you prepare for your test.

How to prepare for your Chapter Test:

☐ **Write down any details that your instructor shares about the test.**
In addition to items such as location, date, time, and essentials to bring, be sure to listen carefully for specific information about the topics covered. Communicate with your instructor concerning any details that may be unclear to you.

☐ **Read the Chapter Summary that begins on page 477 of your textbook.**
Study the appropriate sections in the Chapter Summary. This summary contains the most important material in each section including, definitions, concepts, procedures, and examples.

☐ **Review your *Learning Guide*.**
Go back through the *Solved Problems* and *Pencil Problems* in this chapter of your *Learning Guide*. You may find it helpful to cover up solutions and work through the problems again.

☐ **Study your notes and homework.**
Read through your class notes that you took during this unit, and review the corresponding homework assignments.

☐ **Review quizzes and other feedback from your professor.**
Review any quizzes you have taken and be sure you understand any errors that you made. Seek help with any concepts that are still unclear.

☐ **Complete the Review Exercises that begin on page 479 of your textbook.**
Work the assigned problems from the Review Exercises. These exercises represent the most significant problems for each of the chapter's sections. The answers for all Review Exercises are in the back of your textbook.

☐ **Take the Chapter Test that begins on page 480 of your textbook.**
- Find a quiet place to take the Chapter Test.
- Do not use notes, index cards, or any resources other than those your instructor will allow during the actual test.
- After completing the entire test, check your answers in the back of the textbook.
- Watch the *Chapter Test Prep Video* to review any exercises you may have missed.

       Copyright © 2017 Pearson Education, Inc.

Chapter 7.R Rational Expressions
Integrated Review

Learning Objectives
1. Reduce or simplify fractions.
2. Multiply fractions.
3. Divide fractions.
4. Add and subtract fractions with identical denominators.
5. Add and subtract fractions with unlike denominators.

Learning Objective #1: Reduce or simplify fractions.

✔ *Solved Problem #1* 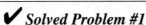 *Pencil Problem #1*

1a. Write $\dfrac{10}{15}$ in simplest form.

$$\dfrac{10}{15} = \dfrac{2 \cdot 5}{3 \cdot 5}$$

$$= \dfrac{2 \cdot \cancel{5}}{3 \cdot \cancel{5}}$$

$$= \dfrac{2}{3}$$

1a. Write $\dfrac{21}{49}$ in simplest form.

1b. Write $-\dfrac{30}{42}$ in simplest form.

$$-\dfrac{30}{42} = -\dfrac{2 \cdot 3 \cdot 5}{2 \cdot 3 \cdot 7}$$

$$= -\dfrac{\cancel{2} \cdot \cancel{3} \cdot 5}{\cancel{2} \cdot \cancel{3} \cdot 7}$$

$$= -\dfrac{5}{7} \text{ or } \dfrac{-5}{7} \text{ or } \dfrac{5}{-7}$$

1b. Write $-\dfrac{108}{60}$ in simplest form.

1c. Write $\dfrac{14x^3}{42x^5}$ in simplest form. Assume that all variable factors in the denominators are not equal to zero.

$$\dfrac{14x^3}{42x^5} = \dfrac{2 \cdot 7 \cdot x \cdot x \cdot x}{2 \cdot 3 \cdot 7 \cdot x \cdot x \cdot x \cdot x \cdot x}$$

$$= \dfrac{1 \cdot \cancel{2} \cdot \cancel{7} \cdot \cancel{x} \cdot \cancel{x} \cdot \cancel{x}}{\cancel{2} \cdot 3 \cdot \cancel{7} \cdot \cancel{x} \cdot \cancel{x} \cdot \cancel{x} \cdot x \cdot x}$$

$$= \dfrac{1}{3x^2}$$

1c. Write $\dfrac{28(x+1)}{60(x+1)^2}$ in simplest form. Assume that all variable factors in the denominators are not equal to zero.

Copyright © 2017 Pearson Education, Inc.

1d. Write $\dfrac{72}{90}$ in simplest form by using the greatest common factor of 72 and 90.

$72 = 2^3 \cdot 3^2$

$90 = 2 \cdot 5 \cdot 3^2$

Greatest Common Factor is $2 \cdot 3^2$ or 18.

$\dfrac{72}{90} = \dfrac{72 \div 18}{90 \div 18}$

$\phantom{\dfrac{72}{90}} = \dfrac{4}{5}$

1d. Write $\dfrac{60}{150}$ in simplest form by using the greatest common factor of 60 and 150.

Learning Objective #2: Multiply fractions.

✔ **Solved Problem #2**

2a. Multiply $\dfrac{x}{8} \cdot \dfrac{10x}{y}$. Assume that all variable factors in the denominators are not equal to zero.

2 is a common factor of 8 and 10. Divide each by 2.

$\dfrac{x}{8} \cdot \dfrac{10x}{y} = \dfrac{x}{\underset{4}{\cancel{8}}} \cdot \dfrac{\overset{5}{\cancel{10}}x}{y}$

$\phantom{\dfrac{x}{8} \cdot \dfrac{10x}{y}} = \dfrac{x \cdot 5x}{4 \cdot y}$

$\phantom{\dfrac{x}{8} \cdot \dfrac{10x}{y}} = \dfrac{5x^2}{4y}$

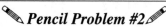 **Pencil Problem #2**

2a. Multiply $\dfrac{x}{4} \cdot \dfrac{y}{3}$. Assume that all variable factors in the denominators are not equal to zero.

Copyright © 2017 Pearson Education, Inc.

2b. Multiply $\dfrac{12x}{y} \cdot \dfrac{y^3}{15x^2}$ Assume that all variable factors in the denominators are not equal to zero.

3 is a common factor of 12 and 15. Divide each by 3. Also, divide numerators and denominators by other common factors, x and y.

$$\frac{12x}{y} \cdot \frac{y^3}{15x^2} = \frac{12x}{y} \cdot \frac{y \cdot y \cdot y}{15x \cdot x}$$

$$= \frac{\overset{4}{\cancel{12}}\,\overset{1}{\cancel{x}}}{\cancel{y}} \cdot \frac{\overset{1}{\cancel{y}} \cdot y \cdot y}{\underset{5}{\cancel{15}}\,\underset{1}{\cancel{x}} \cdot x}$$

$$= \frac{4 \cdot y \cdot y}{5x}$$

$$= \frac{4y^2}{5x}$$

2b. Multiply $\dfrac{10x^2}{y} \cdot \dfrac{y^3}{15x}$. Assume that all variable factors in the denominators are not equal to zero.

Learning Objective #3: Divide fractions.

✔ Solved Problem #3

3a. Divide $\dfrac{6x^2}{y^3} \div \dfrac{4x}{y^2}$.

Assume that variable factors do not cause any denominators to equal zero.

$$\frac{6x^2}{y^3} \div \frac{4x}{y^2} = \frac{6x^2}{y^3} \cdot \frac{y^2}{4x}$$

$$= \frac{\overset{3}{\cancel{6}}\,\overset{1}{\cancel{x}} \cdot x}{\cancel{y} \cdot \cancel{y} \cdot y} \cdot \frac{\overset{1}{\cancel{y}} \cdot \overset{1}{\cancel{y}}}{\underset{2}{\cancel{4}}\,\underset{1}{\cancel{x}}}$$

$$= \frac{3x}{2y}$$

✎ Pencil Problem #3✎

3a. Divide $\dfrac{x^2}{15} \div \dfrac{x}{18}$.

Assume that variable factors do not cause any denominators to equal zero.

3b. Divide $\dfrac{6y}{7z} \div (-15yz)$.

Assume that variable factors do not cause any denominators to equal zero.

$$\dfrac{6y}{7z} \div (-15yz) = -\dfrac{6y}{7z} \cdot \dfrac{1}{15yz}$$

$$= -\dfrac{\overset{2}{\cancel{6}}\,\overset{1}{\cancel{y}}}{7z} \cdot \dfrac{1}{\underset{5}{\cancel{15}}\,\underset{1}{\cancel{y}}\,z}$$

$$= -\dfrac{2}{35z^2}$$

3b. Divide $\left(-\dfrac{x^2 y}{z}\right) \div \left(\dfrac{xy^2}{z^3}\right)$.

Assume that variable factors do not cause any denominators to equal zero.

| **Learning Objective #4:** Add and subtract fractions with identical denominators. |

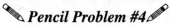 **Solved Problem #4**   **Pencil Problem #4**

4a. Add $\dfrac{2}{13} + \dfrac{5}{13}$.

4a. Add $\dfrac{1}{10} + \dfrac{3}{10}$.

$$\dfrac{2}{13} + \dfrac{5}{13} = \dfrac{2+5}{13}$$

$$= \dfrac{7}{13}$$

Copyright © 2017 Pearson Education, Inc.

4b. Add $\dfrac{1}{17}+\dfrac{10}{17}+\dfrac{12}{17}$.

$$\dfrac{1}{17}+\dfrac{10}{17}+\dfrac{12}{17}=\dfrac{1+10+12}{17}$$
$$=\dfrac{23}{17}$$
$$=1\dfrac{6}{17}$$

4b. Add $\dfrac{7}{8}+\left(-\dfrac{1}{8}\right)$.

> **Learning Objective #5:** Add and subtract fractions with unlike denominators.

✔ Solved Problem #5

5a. Write $\dfrac{2}{3}$ as an equivalent fraction with a denominator of 21.

To obtain a denominator of 21, we must multiply the denominator of the given fraction, $\dfrac{2}{3}$ by 7.

So that we do not change the value of the fraction, we also multiply the numerator by 7.

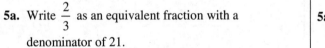

$$\dfrac{2}{3}=\dfrac{2\cdot 7}{3\cdot 7}=\dfrac{14}{21}$$

✎ Pencil Problem #5 ✎

5a. Write $\dfrac{3}{4}$ as an equivalent fraction with a denominator of 20.

5b. Add $\dfrac{1}{2}+\dfrac{3}{5}$.

$2 = 2 \cdot 1$
$5 = 1 \cdot 5$
Least Common Multiple is $2 \cdot 5$ or 10.
We rewrite both fractions as equivalent fractions with the least common denominator, 10, then perform the operation.

$$\frac{1}{2}+\frac{3}{5} = \frac{1 \cdot 5}{2 \cdot 5}+\frac{3 \cdot 2}{5 \cdot 2}$$
$$= \frac{5}{10}+\frac{6}{10}$$
$$= \frac{11}{10} = 1\frac{1}{10}$$

5b. Add $\dfrac{5}{24}+\dfrac{7}{30}$.

5c. Subtract $\dfrac{7}{12}-\dfrac{3}{10}$.

$12 = 2^2 \cdot 3$
$10 = 2 \cdot 5$

Least Common Multiple is $2^2 \cdot 3 \cdot 5$ or 60.
We rewrite both fractions as equivalent fractions with the least common denominator, 60, then perform the operation.

$$\frac{7}{12}-\frac{3}{10} = \frac{7 \cdot 5}{12 \cdot 5}-\frac{3 \cdot 6}{10 \cdot 6}$$
$$= \frac{35}{60}-\frac{18}{60}$$
$$= \frac{35-18}{60} = \frac{17}{60}$$

5c. Subtract $\dfrac{13}{18}-\dfrac{2}{9}$.

Answers for Pencil Problems:

1a. $\dfrac{3}{7}$ **1b.** $-\dfrac{9}{5}$ **1c.** $\dfrac{7}{15(x+1)}$ **1d.** $\dfrac{2}{5}$ **2a.** $\dfrac{xy}{12}$ **2b.** $\dfrac{2xy^2}{3}$ **3a.** $\dfrac{6x}{5}$ **3b.** $-\dfrac{xz^2}{y}$ **4a.** $\dfrac{2}{5}$ **4b.** $\dfrac{3}{4}$

5a. $\dfrac{15}{20}$ **5b.** $\dfrac{53}{120}$ **5c.** $\dfrac{1}{2}$

Copyright © 2017 Pearson Education, Inc.

Section 7.1
Rational Expressions and Their Simplification

Ouch! That Hurts!!

Though it may not be fun to get a flu shot,
it is a great way to protect yourself from getting sick!

In this section of the textbook, one of the application problems will explore the costs for inoculating various percentages of the population.

First Steps:

☐ **Take comprehensive notes** from your instructor's lecture and insert your notes into this section of the *Learning Guide*. Be sure to write down all examples, definitions, and other key concepts. Additional learning resources include the *Video Lecture Series*, the *PowerPoints*, and Section 7.1 of your textbook which begins on page 484.

☐ Complete the *Concept and Vocabulary Check* on page 491 of the textbook.

Guided Practice:

☐ Review each of the following *Solved Problems* and complete each *Pencil Problem*.

Learning Objective #1: Find numbers for which a rational expression is undefined.

✔ *Solved Problem #1*	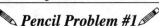 *Pencil Problem #1*
1a. Find all the numbers for which the rational expression is undefined: $$\frac{7x-28}{8x-40}$$	**1a.** Find all the numbers for which the rational expression is undefined: $$\frac{13}{5x-20}$$

A rational expression is undefined when its denominator is equal to 0.

Set the denominator equal to 0 and solve for x.

$$8x - 40 = 0$$
$$8x = 40$$
$$x = 5$$

The rational expression is undefined for $x = 5$.

1b. Find all the numbers for which the rational expression is undefined:

$$\frac{8x - 40}{x^2 + 3x - 28}$$

Set the denominator equal to 0 and solve for x.

$$x^2 + 3x - 28 = 0$$
$$(x + 7)(x - 4) = 0$$

$$x + 7 = 0 \quad \text{or} \quad x - 4 = 0$$
$$x = -7 \qquad\qquad x = 4$$

The rational expression is undefined for $x = -7$ and $x = 4$.

1b. Find all the numbers for which the rational expression is undefined:

$$\frac{y + 5}{y^2 - 25}$$

Learning Objective #2: Simplify rational expressions.

✔ **Solved Problem #2**

2a. Simplify: $\dfrac{7x + 28}{21x}$

Factor the numerator and denominator.
$$\frac{7x + 28}{21x} = \frac{7(x + 4)}{7 \cdot 3x}$$

Divide out common factors.
$$\frac{7x + 28}{21x} = \frac{7(x + 4)}{7 \cdot 3x}$$
$$= \frac{x + 4}{3x}$$

✎ **Pencil Problem #2** ✎

2a. Simplify: $\dfrac{5x - 15}{25}$

2b. Simplify: $\dfrac{x^3 - x^2}{7x - 7}$

Factor the numerator and denominator.
$$\frac{x^3 - x^2}{7x - 7} = \frac{x^2(x - 1)}{7(x - 1)}$$

Divide out common factors.
$$\frac{x^3 - x^2}{7x - 7} = \frac{x^2(x - 1)}{7(x - 1)}$$
$$= \frac{x^2}{7}$$

2b. Simplify: $\dfrac{2x + 3}{2x + 5}$

Copyright © 2017 Pearson Education, Inc.

2c. Simplify: $\dfrac{x^2-1}{x^2+2x+1}$

2c. Simplify: $\dfrac{4x-8}{x^2-4x+4}$

Factor the numerator and denominator.

$$\frac{x^2-1}{x^2+2x+1} = \frac{(x+1)(x-1)}{(x+1)^2}$$

Divide out common factors.

$$\frac{x^2-1}{x^2+2x+1} = \frac{(x+1)(x-1)}{(x+1)^2}$$

$$= \frac{\cancel{(x+1)}(x-1)}{\cancel{(x+1)}(x+1)}$$

$$= \frac{x-1}{x+1}$$

2d. Simplify: $\dfrac{9x^2-49}{28-12x}$

2d. Simplify: $\dfrac{y^2-y-12}{4-y}$

Factor the numerator and denominator.

$$\frac{9x^2-49}{28-12x} = \frac{(3x+7)(3x-7)}{4(7-3x)}$$

Divide out common factors.
Notice that $(3x-7)$ and $(7-3x)$ are opposites and, therefore, their division results in -1.

$$\frac{9x^2-49}{28-12x} = \frac{(3x+7)(3x-7)}{4(7-3x)}$$

$$= \frac{(3x+7)\overset{-1}{\cancel{(3x-7)}}}{4\,\cancel{(7-3x)}}$$

$$= \frac{-(3x+7)}{4} \quad \text{or} \quad -\frac{3x+7}{4} \quad \text{or} \quad \frac{-3x-7}{4}$$

Copyright © 2017 Pearson Education, Inc.

Learning Objective #3: Solve applied problems involving rational expressions.

✔ **Solved Problem #3**	✎ **Pencil Problem #3** ✎

3. The cost, y, in millions of dollars, to remove x percent of the pollutants that are discharged into a river is given by the equation $y = \dfrac{250x}{100-x}$.

3a. Find the cost to remove 40% of the pollutants.

$y = \dfrac{250x}{100-x}$

$y = \dfrac{250(40)}{100-40} \approx 167$

The cost is approximately $167 million.

3b. Find the cost to remove 95% of the pollutants.

$y = \dfrac{250x}{100-x}$

$y = \dfrac{250(95)}{100-95} = 4750$

The cost is approximately $4750 million or $4.75 billion.

3c. For what value of x is the expression undefined?

Set the denominator equal to 0.

$0 = 100 - x$

$x = 100$

The expression undefined when $x = 100$.

---

3. A company that manufactures bicycles has costs given by the equation $C = \dfrac{100x + 100,000}{x}$, in which x is the number of bicycles manufactured and C is the cost to manufacture each bicycle.

3a. Find the cost per bicycle when manufacturing 500 bicycles.

3b. Find the cost per bicycle when manufacturing 4000 bicycles.

3c. Does the cost per bicycle increase or decrease as more bicycles are manufactured?

Answers for Pencil Problems (*Textbook Exercise references in parentheses*):

1a. $x = 4$ *(7.1 #5)*   **1b.** $y = -5$ and $y = 5$ *(7.1 #17)*

2a. $\dfrac{x-3}{5}$ *(7.1 #23)*   **2b.** cannot be simplified *(7.1 #45)*   **2c.** $\dfrac{4}{x-2}$ *(7.1 #39)*   **2d.** $-y - 3$ *(7.1 #71)*

3a. $300   *(7.1 #89)*   **3b.** $125   *(7.1 #89)*   **3c.** decrease *(7.1 #89)*

Homework:

☐ **Review the Section 7.1 summary** on page 557 of the textbook.

☐ **Insert your homework** into this section of the *Learning Guide*. Show all work neatly and check your answers. Strive to work through difficulties when possible, making note of any exercises where you need additional help. Remember, even if your instructor assigns homework through *MyMathLab*, you should still write out your work.

    Copyright © 2017 Pearson Education, Inc.

Section 7.2
Multiplying and Dividing Rational Expressions

Where Did the Numbers Go???

When learning algebra, students often long for the days when the math that they were doing only involved numbers.

It can be quite helpful to recognize that algebraic techniques follow the same underlying principles as their corresponding numeric techniques.

In this section of the textbook, you should notice that we multiply rational expressions in the same way that we multiply rational numbers.

First Steps:

☐ **Take comprehensive notes** from your instructor's lecture and insert your notes into this section of the *Learning Guide*. Be sure to write down all examples, definitions, and other key concepts. Additional learning resources include the *Video Lecture Series*, the *PowerPoints*, and Section 7.2 of your textbook which begins on page 494.

☐ Complete the *Concept and Vocabulary Check* on page 498 of the textbook.

Guided Practice:

☐ Review each of the following *Solved Problems* and complete each *Pencil Problem*.

Learning Objective #1: Multiply rational expressions.

✔ *Solved Problem #1*	✎ *Pencil Problem #1*✎
1a. Multiply: $\dfrac{9}{x+4} \cdot \dfrac{x-5}{2}$	**1a.** Multiply: $\dfrac{4}{x+3} \cdot \dfrac{x-5}{9}$

$$\frac{9}{x+4} \cdot \frac{x-5}{2} = \frac{9(x-5)}{(x+4)2}$$
$$= \frac{9x-45}{2x+8}$$

Copyright © 2017 Pearson Education, Inc.

1b. Multiply: $\dfrac{x+4}{x-7} \cdot \dfrac{3x-21}{8x+32}$

$\dfrac{x+4}{x-7} \cdot \dfrac{3x-21}{8x+32} = \dfrac{x+4}{x-7} \cdot \dfrac{3(x-7)}{8(x+4)}$

$= \dfrac{\cancel{x+4}}{\cancel{x-7}} \cdot \dfrac{3\,\cancel{(x-7)}}{8\,\cancel{(x+4)}}$

$= \dfrac{3}{8}$

1b. Multiply: $\dfrac{x-3}{x+5} \cdot \dfrac{4x+20}{9x-27}$

1c. Multiply: $\dfrac{x-5}{x-2} \cdot \dfrac{x^2-4}{9x-45}$

$\dfrac{x-5}{x-2} \cdot \dfrac{x^2-4}{9x-45} = \dfrac{x-5}{x-2} \cdot \dfrac{(x+2)(x-2)}{9(x-5)}$

$= \dfrac{\cancel{x-5}}{\cancel{x-2}} \cdot \dfrac{(x+2)\,\cancel{(x-2)}}{9\,\cancel{(x-5)}}$

$= \dfrac{x+2}{9}$

1c. Multiply: $\dfrac{x^2-25}{x^2-3x-10} \cdot \dfrac{x+2}{x}$

1d. Multiply: $\dfrac{5x+5}{7x-7x^2} \cdot \dfrac{2x^2+x-3}{4x^2-9}$

$\dfrac{5x+5}{7x-7x^2} \cdot \dfrac{2x^2+x-3}{4x^2-9} = \dfrac{5(x+1)}{7x(1-x)} \cdot \dfrac{(2x+3)(x-1)}{(2x+3)(2x-3)}$

$= \dfrac{5(x+1)}{7x\cancel{(1-x)}} \cdot \dfrac{\cancel{(2x+3)}\,\overset{-1}{\cancel{(x-1)}}}{\cancel{(2x+3)}(2x-3)}$

$= \dfrac{-5(x+1)}{7x(2x-3)} \quad \text{or} \quad -\dfrac{5(x+1)}{7x(2x-3)}$

1d. Multiply: $\dfrac{25-y^2}{y^2-2y-35} \cdot \dfrac{y^2-8y-20}{y^2-3y-10}$

Copyright © 2017 Pearson Education, Inc.

Learning Objective #2: Divide rational expressions.

✔ Solved Problem #2

2a. Divide: $(x+3) \div \dfrac{x-4}{x+7}$

$$(x+3) \div \frac{x-4}{x+7} = \frac{x+3}{1} \cdot \frac{x+7}{x-4}$$
$$= \frac{(x+3)(x+7)}{x-4}$$

✎ Pencil Problem #2 ✎

2a. Divide: $\dfrac{15}{x} \div \dfrac{3}{2x}$

2b. Divide: $\dfrac{x^2+5x+6}{x^2-25} \div \dfrac{x+2}{x+5}$

$$\frac{x^2+5x+6}{x^2-25} \div \frac{x+2}{x+5} = \frac{x^2+5x+6}{x^2-25} \cdot \frac{x+5}{x+2}$$
$$= \frac{(x+3)(x+2)}{(x+5)(x-5)} \cdot \frac{x+5}{x+2}$$
$$= \frac{(x+3)\cancel{(x+2)}}{\cancel{(x+5)}(x-5)} \cdot \frac{\cancel{x+5}}{\cancel{x+2}}$$
$$= \frac{x+3}{x-5}$$

2b. Divide: $\dfrac{x^2-4}{x} \div \dfrac{x+2}{x-2}$

Copyright © 2017 Pearson Education, Inc.

2c. Divide: $\dfrac{y^2+3y+2}{y^2+1} \div \left(5y^2+10y\right)$

2c. Divide: $\left(y^2-16\right) \div \dfrac{y^2+3y-4}{y^2+4}$

$\dfrac{y^2+3y+2}{y^2+1} \div \left(5y^2+10y\right) = \dfrac{y^2+3y+2}{y^2+1} \div \dfrac{5y^2+10y}{1}$

$= \dfrac{y^2+3y+2}{y^2+1} \cdot \dfrac{1}{5y^2+10y}$

$= \dfrac{(y+2)(y+1)}{y^2+1} \cdot \dfrac{1}{5y(y+2)}$

$= \dfrac{\cancel{(y+2)}(y+1)}{y^2+1} \cdot \dfrac{1}{5y\cancel{(y+2)}}$

$= \dfrac{y+1}{5y(y^2+1)}$

Answers for Pencil Problems *(Textbook Exercise references in parentheses)*:

1a. $\dfrac{4x-20}{9x+27}$ *(7.2 #1)*   **1b.** $\dfrac{4}{9}$ *(7.2 #7)*   **1c.** $\dfrac{x+5}{x}$ *(7.2 #11)*   **1d.** $\dfrac{-(y-10)}{y-7}$ or $-\dfrac{y-10}{y-7}$ *(7.2 #27)*

2a. 10 *(7.2 #37)*   **2b.** $\dfrac{(x-2)^2}{x}$ *(7.2 #43)*   **2c.** $\dfrac{(y-4)(y^2+4)}{y-1}$ *(7.2 #45)*

Homework:

☐ **Review the Section 7.2 summary** on page 558 of the textbook.

☐ **Insert your homework** into this section of the *Learning Guide*. Show all work neatly and check your answers. Strive to work through difficulties when possible, making note of any exercises where you need additional help. Remember, even if your instructor assigns homework through *MyMathLab*, you should still write out your work.

Copyright © 2017 Pearson Education, Inc.

Section 7.3
Adding and Subtracting Rational Expressions
with the Same Denominator

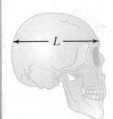 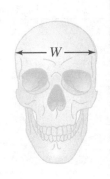

Digging Up the Past!!

Anthropologists and forensic scientists classify skulls as "long," "medium," and "round."

To make this determination they use a mathematical expression that involves a skull's length, *L*, and width, *W*, as shown here.

When you work the exercises in the textbook, you will explore this expression, and use it to classify a skull that is 5 inches wide and 6 inches long.

First Steps:

☐ **Take comprehensive notes** from your instructor's lecture and insert your notes into this section of the *Learning Guide*. Be sure to write down all examples, definitions, and other key concepts. Additional learning resources include the *Video Lecture Series*, the *PowerPoints*, and Section 7.3 of your textbook which begins on page 501.

☐ Complete the *Concept and Vocabulary Check* on page 506 of the textbook.

Guided Practice:

☐ Review each of the following *Solved Problems* and complete each *Pencil Problem*.

Learning Objective #1: Add rational expressions with the same denominator.

✔ **Solved Problem #1**

1a. Add: $\dfrac{3x-2}{5}+\dfrac{2x+12}{5}$

$$\dfrac{3x-2}{5}+\dfrac{2x+12}{5}=\dfrac{3x-2+2x+12}{5}$$

$$=\dfrac{5x+10}{5}$$

$$=\dfrac{\overset{1}{\cancel{5}}(x+2)}{\underset{1}{\cancel{5}}}$$

$$=x+2$$

✎ **Pencil Problem #1** ✎

1a. Add: $\dfrac{x-3}{12}+\dfrac{5x+21}{12}$

1b. Add: $\dfrac{x^2}{x^2-25}+\dfrac{25-10x}{x^2-25}$

$$\dfrac{x^2}{x^2-25}+\dfrac{25-10x}{x^2-25}=\dfrac{x^2-10x+25}{x^2-25}$$

$$=\dfrac{(x-5)^2}{(x+5)(x-5)}$$

$$=\dfrac{(x-5)\,\cancel{(x-5)}}{(x+5)\,\cancel{(x-5)}}$$

$$=\dfrac{x-5}{x+5}$$

1b. Add: $\dfrac{x^2-2}{x^2+x-2}+\dfrac{2x-x^2}{x^2+x-2}$

Learning Objective #2: Subtract rational expressions with the same denominator.

✔ **Solved Problem #2**

✎ **Pencil Problem #2** ✎

2a. Subtract: $\dfrac{4x+5}{x+7}-\dfrac{x}{x+7}$

$$\dfrac{4x+5}{x+7}-\dfrac{x}{x+7}=\dfrac{4x+5-x}{x+7}$$

$$=\dfrac{3x+5}{x+7}$$

2a. Subtract: $\dfrac{3x}{5x-4}-\dfrac{4}{5x-4}$

2b. Subtract: $\dfrac{3x^2+4x}{x-1}-\dfrac{11x-4}{x-1}$

$$\dfrac{3x^2+4x}{x-1}-\dfrac{11x-4}{x-1}=\dfrac{3x^2+4x-(11x-4)}{x-1}$$

$$=\dfrac{3x^2+4x-11x+4}{x-1}$$

$$=\dfrac{3x^2-7x+4}{x-1}$$

$$=\dfrac{(3x-4)(x-1)}{x-1}$$

$$=3x-4$$

2b. Subtract: $\dfrac{4x}{4x-3}-\dfrac{3}{4x-3}$

Copyright © 2017 Pearson Education, Inc.

2c. Subtract: $\dfrac{y^2+3y-6}{y^2-5y+4}-\dfrac{4y-4-2y^2}{y^2-5y+4}$

$$\dfrac{y^2+3y-6}{y^2-5y+4}-\dfrac{4y-4-2y^2}{y^2-5y+4}=\dfrac{y^2+3y-6-(4y-4-2y^2)}{y^2-5y+4}$$

$$=\dfrac{y^2+3y-6-4y+4+2y^2}{y^2-5y+4}$$

$$=\dfrac{3y^2-y-2}{y^2-5y+4}$$

$$=\dfrac{(3y+2)(y-1)}{(y-4)(y-1)}$$

$$=\dfrac{3y+2}{y-4}$$

2c. Subtract: $\dfrac{4y^2+5}{9y^2-64}-\dfrac{y^2-y+29}{9y^2-64}$

Learning Objective #3: Add and subtract rational expressions with opposite denominators.

✔ *Solved Problem #3*

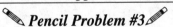 *Pencil Problem #3*

3a. Add: $\dfrac{x^2}{x-7}+\dfrac{4x+21}{7-x}$

$$\dfrac{x^2}{x-7}+\dfrac{4x+21}{7-x}=\dfrac{x^2}{x-7}+\dfrac{(-1)}{(-1)}\cdot\dfrac{4x+21}{7-x}$$

$$=\dfrac{x^2}{x-7}+\dfrac{-4x-21}{x-7}$$

$$=\dfrac{x^2-4x-21}{x-7}$$

$$=\dfrac{(x+3)(x-7)}{x-7}$$

$$=x+3$$

3a. Add: $\dfrac{6x+7}{x-6}+\dfrac{3x}{6-x}$

3b. Subtract: $\dfrac{7x - x^2}{x^2 - 2x - 9} - \dfrac{5x - 3x^2}{9 + 2x - x^2}$

$$\dfrac{7x - x^2}{x^2 - 2x - 9} - \dfrac{5x - 3x^2}{9 + 2x - x^2} = \dfrac{7x - x^2}{x^2 - 2x - 9} - \dfrac{3x^2 - 5x}{x^2 - 2x - 9}$$

$$= \dfrac{7x - x^2 - (3x^2 - 5x)}{x^2 - 2x - 9}$$

$$= \dfrac{7x - x^2 - 3x^2 + 5x}{x^2 - 2x - 9}$$

$$= \dfrac{-4x^2 + 12x}{x^2 - 2x - 9}$$

3b. Subtract: $\dfrac{x - 2}{x^2 - 25} - \dfrac{x - 2}{25 - x^2}$

Answers for Pencil Problems (*Textbook Exercise references in parentheses*):

1a. $\dfrac{x + 3}{2}$ *(7.3 #5)* **1b.** $\dfrac{2}{x + 2}$ *(7.3 #21)*

2a. $\dfrac{3x - 4}{5x - 4}$ *(7.3 #25)* **2b.** 1 *(7.3 #27)* **2c.** $\dfrac{y + 3}{3y + 8}$ *(7.3 #35)*

3a. $\dfrac{3x + 7}{x - 6}$ *(7.3 #41)* **3b.** $\dfrac{2x - 4}{x^2 - 25}$ *(7.3 #57)*

Homework:

☐ **Review the Section 7.3 summary** on page 558 of the textbook.

☐ **Insert your homework** into this section of the *Learning Guide*. Show all work neatly and check your answers. Strive to work through difficulties when possible, making note of any exercises where you need additional help. Remember, even if your instructor assigns homework through *MyMathLab*, you should still write out your work.

Copyright © 2017 Pearson Education, Inc.

Section 7.4
Adding and Subtracting Rational Expressions
with Different Denominators

> ### Is There a Doctor in the House?
>
> In this section's exercise set, you will use two formulas that model drug dosage for children. Before working with these models, we continue drawing on your experience from arithmetic to add and subtract rational expressions that have different denominators.

First Steps:

☐ **Take comprehensive notes** from your instructor's lecture and insert your notes into this section of the *Learning Guide*. Be sure to write down all examples, definitions, and other key concepts. Additional learning resources include the *Video Lecture Series*, the *PowerPoints*, and Section 7.4 of your textbook which begins on page 509.

☐ Complete the *Concept and Vocabulary Check* on page 516 of the textbook.

Guided Practice:

☐ Review each of the following *Solved Problems* and complete each *Pencil Problem*.

Learning Objective #1: Find the least common denominator.	
✔ *Solved Problem #1*	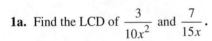 *Pencil Problem #1*

1a. Find the LCD of $\dfrac{3}{10x^2}$ and $\dfrac{7}{15x}$.

List the factors for each denominator.
$10x^2 = 2 \cdot 5x^2$
$15x = 3 \cdot 5x$

LCD $= 2 \cdot 3 \cdot 5 \cdot x^2 = 30x^2$

1a. Find the LCD of $\dfrac{8}{15x^2}$ and $\dfrac{5}{6x^5}$.

1b. Find the LCD of $\dfrac{2}{x+3}$ and $\dfrac{4}{x-3}$.

List the factors for each denominator.
$x+3 = 1(x+3)$
$x-3 = 1(x-3)$

LCD $= (x+3)(x-3)$

1b. Find the LCD of $\dfrac{4}{x-3}$ and $\dfrac{7}{x+1}$.

1c. Find the LCD of $\dfrac{9}{7x^2 + 28x}$ and $\dfrac{11}{x^2 + 8x + 16}$.

List the factors for each denominator.

$7x^2 + 28x = 7x(x + 4)$

$x^2 + 8x + 16 = (x + 4)^2$

LCD $= 7x(x + 4)^2$

1c. Find the LCD of $\dfrac{7}{y^2 - 1}$ and $\dfrac{y}{y^2 - 2y + 1}$.

Learning Objective #2: Add and subtract rational expressions with different denominators.

✔ **Solved Problem #2**

2a. Add: $\dfrac{3}{10x^2} + \dfrac{7}{15x}$

LCD $= 30x^2$

$\dfrac{3}{10x^2} + \dfrac{7}{15x} = \dfrac{3}{3} \cdot \dfrac{3}{10x^2} + \dfrac{2x}{2x} \cdot \dfrac{7}{15x}$

$= \dfrac{9}{30x^2} + \dfrac{14x}{30x^2}$

$= \dfrac{9 + 14x}{30x^2}$

✏ **Pencil Problem #2** ✏

2a. Add: $\dfrac{4}{x} + \dfrac{7}{2x^2}$

2b. Add: $\dfrac{2}{x+3} + \dfrac{4}{x-3}$

LCD $= (x+3)(x-3)$

$\dfrac{2}{x+3} + \dfrac{4}{x-3} = \dfrac{x-3}{x-3} \cdot \dfrac{2}{x+3} + \dfrac{x+3}{x+3} \cdot \dfrac{4}{x-3}$

$= \dfrac{2x-6}{(x+3)(x-3)} + \dfrac{4x+12}{(x+3)(x-3)}$

$= \dfrac{2x-6+4x+12}{(x+3)(x-3)}$

$= \dfrac{6x+6}{(x+3)(x-3)}$

2b. Add: $\dfrac{4}{x} + \dfrac{3}{x-5}$

Copyright © 2017 Pearson Education, Inc.

2c. Subtract: $\dfrac{x}{x+5}-1$

LCD = $x+5$

$$\dfrac{x}{x+5}-1 = \dfrac{x}{x+5}-\dfrac{x+5}{x+5}$$
$$= \dfrac{x-(x+5)}{x+5}$$
$$= \dfrac{x-x-5}{x+5}$$
$$= \dfrac{-5}{x+5} \ \text{ or } \ -\dfrac{5}{x+5}$$

2c. Subtract: $\dfrac{x}{x+7}-1$

2d. Subtract: $\dfrac{5}{y^2-5y}-\dfrac{y}{5y-25}$

Factor the denominators.

$$\dfrac{5}{y^2-5y}-\dfrac{y}{5y-25} = \dfrac{5}{y(y-5)}-\dfrac{y}{5(y-5)}$$

LCD = $5y(y-5)$

$$\dfrac{5}{y^2-5y}-\dfrac{y}{5y-25} = \dfrac{5}{y(y-5)}-\dfrac{y}{5(y-5)}$$
$$= \dfrac{5}{5}\cdot\dfrac{5}{y(y-5)}-\dfrac{y}{y}\cdot\dfrac{y}{5(y-5)}$$
$$= \dfrac{25}{5y(y-5)}-\dfrac{y^2}{5y(y-5)}$$
$$= \dfrac{25-y^2}{5y(y-5)}$$
$$= \dfrac{(5+y)(5-y)}{5y(y-5)}$$
$$= \dfrac{(5+y)\overset{-1}{\cancel{(5-y)}}}{5y\underset{1}{\cancel{(y-5)}}}$$
$$= -\dfrac{5+y}{5y}$$

2d. Subtract: $\dfrac{2x+9}{x^2-7x+12}-\dfrac{2}{x-3}$

2e. Add: $\dfrac{4x}{x^2-25}+\dfrac{3}{5-x}$

2e. Add: $\dfrac{3}{x^2-1}+\dfrac{4}{(x+1)^2}$

Factor the denominators.

$$\frac{4x}{x^2-25}+\frac{3}{5-x}=\frac{4x}{(x+5)(x-5)}+\frac{3}{5-x}$$

LCD $=(x+5)(x-5)$

$$\frac{4x}{x^2-25}+\frac{3}{5-x}=\frac{4x}{(x+5)(x-5)}+\frac{3}{5-x}$$

$$=\frac{4x}{(x+5)(x-5)}+\frac{-1(x+5)}{-1(x+5)}\cdot\frac{3}{5-x}$$

$$=\frac{4x}{(x+5)(x-5)}+\frac{-1(x+5)\cdot 3}{(x+5)(x-5)}$$

$$=\frac{4x}{(x+5)(x-5)}+\frac{-3x-15}{(x+5)(x-5)}$$

$$=\frac{4x-3x-15}{(x+5)(x-5)}$$

$$=\frac{x-15}{(x+5)(x-5)}$$

<u>**Answers**</u> for Pencil Problems *(Textbook Exercise references in parentheses)*:

1a. $2\cdot 3\cdot 5\cdot x^5=30x^5$ *(7.4 #3)*   **1b.** $(x-3)(x+1)$ *(7.4 #5)*   **1c.** $(y+1)(y-1)(y-1)$ *(7.4 #13)*

2a. $\dfrac{8x+7}{2x^2}$ *(7.4 #21)*   **2b.** $\dfrac{7x-20}{x(x-5)}$ *(7.4 #29)*   **2c.** $\dfrac{-7}{x+7}$ or $-\dfrac{7}{x+7}$ *(7.4 #35)*

2d. $\dfrac{17}{(x-3)(x-4)}$ *(7.4 #49)*   **2e.** $\dfrac{7x-1}{(x+1)(x+1)(x-1)}$ *(7.4 #51)*

Homework:

☐ **Review the Section 7.4 summary** on page 559 of the textbook.

☐ **Insert your homework** into this section of the *Learning Guide*. Show all work neatly and check your answers. Strive to work through difficulties when possible, making note of any exercises where you need additional help. Remember, even if your instructor assigns homework through *MyMathLab*, you should still write out your work.

   Copyright © 2017 Pearson Education, Inc.

Section 7.5
Complex Rational Expressions

S h o c k i n g ! ! ! ! !

If two electrical resistors are connected in parallel, then the total resistance
in the circuit can be calculated using a complex rational expression.

One of the application exercises in the textbook will guide you through this process.

First Steps:

☐ **Take comprehensive notes** from your instructor's lecture and insert your notes into this section of the *Learning Guide*. Be sure to write down all examples, definitions, and other key concepts. Additional learning resources include the *Video Lecture Series*, the *PowerPoints*, and Section 7.5 of your textbook which begins on page 521.

☐ Complete the *Concept and Vocabulary Check* on page 526 of the textbook.

Guided Practice:

☐ Review each of the following *Solved Problems* and complete each *Pencil Problem*.

Learning Objective #1: Simplifying complex rational expressions by dividing.

✔ *Solved Problem #1*	✎ *Pencil Problem #1* ✎
1a. Simplify: $\dfrac{\dfrac{1}{4}+\dfrac{2}{3}}{\dfrac{2}{3}-\dfrac{1}{4}}$	**1a.** Simplify: $\dfrac{\dfrac{1}{2}+\dfrac{1}{4}}{\dfrac{1}{2}+\dfrac{1}{3}}$

Add to get a single rational expression in the numerator.

$$\frac{1}{4}+\frac{2}{3}=\frac{3}{12}+\frac{8}{12}=\frac{11}{12}$$

Subtract to get a single rational expression in the denominator.

$$\frac{2}{3}-\frac{1}{4}=\frac{8}{12}-\frac{3}{12}=\frac{5}{12}$$

Perform the division indicated by the fraction bar. Invert and multiply.

$$\frac{\dfrac{1}{4}+\dfrac{2}{3}}{\dfrac{2}{3}-\dfrac{1}{4}}=\frac{\dfrac{11}{12}}{\dfrac{5}{12}}=\frac{11}{12}\cdot\frac{12}{5}=\frac{11}{5}$$

1b. Simplify: $\dfrac{2-\dfrac{1}{x}}{2+\dfrac{1}{x}}$

1b. Simplify: $\dfrac{7-\dfrac{2}{x}}{5+\dfrac{1}{x}}$

Subtract to get a single rational expression in the numerator.

$$2-\frac{1}{x}=\frac{2x}{x}-\frac{1}{x}=\frac{2x-1}{x}$$

Add to get a single rational expression in the denominator.

$$2+\frac{1}{x}=\frac{2x}{x}+\frac{1}{x}=\frac{2x+1}{x}$$

Perform the division indicated by the fraction bar. Invert and multiply.

$$\frac{2-\dfrac{1}{x}}{2+\dfrac{1}{x}}=\frac{\dfrac{2x-1}{x}}{\dfrac{2x+1}{x}}$$

$$=\frac{2x-1}{x}\cdot\frac{x}{2x+1}$$

$$=\frac{2x-1}{\cancel{x}}\cdot\frac{\cancel{x}}{2x+1}$$

$$=\frac{2x-1}{2x+1}$$

1c. Simplify: $\dfrac{\dfrac{1}{x}-\dfrac{1}{y}}{\dfrac{1}{xy}}$

1c. Simplify: $\dfrac{x+\dfrac{2}{y}}{\dfrac{x}{y}}$

Subtract to get a single rational expression in the numerator.

$$\frac{1}{x}-\frac{1}{y}=\frac{y}{xy}-\frac{x}{xy}=\frac{y-x}{xy}$$

Perform the division indicated by the fraction bar. Invert and multiply.

$$\frac{\dfrac{y-x}{xy}}{\dfrac{1}{xy}}=\frac{y-x}{xy}\cdot\frac{xy}{1}$$

$$=\frac{y-x}{\cancel{xy}}\cdot\frac{\cancel{xy}}{1}$$

$$=y-x$$

Copyright © 2017 Pearson Education, Inc.

Learning Objective #2: Simplify complex rational expressions by multiplying by the LCD.	
✔ *Solved Problem #2*	✎ *Pencil Problem #2* ✎

2a. Simplify by the LCD method: $\dfrac{\dfrac{1}{4}+\dfrac{2}{3}}{\dfrac{2}{3}-\dfrac{1}{4}}$

Multiply the numerator and the denominator by the LCD of 12.

$$\frac{\dfrac{1}{4}+\dfrac{2}{3}}{\dfrac{2}{3}-\dfrac{1}{4}}=\frac{12\left(\dfrac{1}{4}+\dfrac{2}{3}\right)}{12\left(\dfrac{2}{3}-\dfrac{1}{4}\right)}$$

$$=\frac{12\cdot\dfrac{1}{4}+12\cdot\dfrac{2}{3}}{12\cdot\dfrac{2}{3}-12\cdot\dfrac{1}{4}}$$

$$=\frac{3+8}{8-3}$$

$$=\frac{11}{5}$$

2a. Simplify by the LCD method: $\dfrac{\dfrac{2}{5}-\dfrac{1}{3}}{\dfrac{2}{3}-\dfrac{3}{4}}$

2b. Simplify by the LCD method: $\dfrac{2-\dfrac{1}{x}}{2+\dfrac{1}{x}}$

Multiply the numerator and the denominator by the LCD of x.

$$\frac{2-\dfrac{1}{x}}{2+\dfrac{1}{x}}=\frac{x\left(2-\dfrac{1}{x}\right)}{x\left(2+\dfrac{1}{x}\right)}$$

$$=\frac{x\cdot2-x\cdot\dfrac{1}{x}}{x\cdot2+x\cdot\dfrac{1}{x}}$$

$$=\frac{2x-1}{2x+1}$$

2b. Simplify by the LCD method: $\dfrac{\dfrac{3}{4}-x}{\dfrac{3}{4}+x}$

Copyright © 2017 Pearson Education, Inc.   215

2c. Simplify by the LCD method: $\dfrac{\dfrac{1}{x}-\dfrac{1}{y}}{\dfrac{1}{xy}}$

Multiply the numerator and the denominator by the LCD of xy.

$$\frac{\dfrac{1}{x}-\dfrac{1}{y}}{\dfrac{1}{xy}}=\frac{xy\left(\dfrac{1}{x}-\dfrac{1}{y}\right)}{xy\left(\dfrac{1}{xy}\right)}$$

$$=\frac{xy\cdot\dfrac{1}{x}-xy\cdot\dfrac{1}{y}}{xy\cdot\dfrac{1}{xy}}$$

$$=\frac{y-x}{1}$$

$$=y-x$$

2c. Simplify by the LCD method: $\dfrac{\dfrac{1}{x}+\dfrac{1}{y}}{xy}$

Answers for Pencil Problems *(Textbook Exercise references in parentheses)*:

1a. $\dfrac{9}{10}$ *(7.5 #1)*   **1b.** $\dfrac{7x-2}{5x+1}$ *(7.5 #9)*   **1c.** $\dfrac{xy+2}{x}$ *(7.5 #21)*

2a. $-\dfrac{4}{5}$ *(7.5 #5)*   **2b.** $\dfrac{3-4x}{3+4x}$ *(7.5 #7)*   **2c.** $\dfrac{y+x}{x^2y^2}$ *(7.5 #23)*

Homework:

☐ **Review the Section 7.5 summary** on page 559 of the textbook.

☐ **Insert your homework** into this section of the *Learning Guide*. Show all work neatly and check your answers. Strive to work through difficulties when possible, making note of any exercises where you need additional help. Remember, even if your instructor assigns homework through *MyMathLab*, you should still write out your work.

Copyright © 2017 Pearson Education, Inc.

Section 7.6
Solving Rational Equations

Stock Up !!!!!

Grocery stores want to control costs.
By averaging the costs to purchase soup and to pay storage costs, a particular store owner has determined that the yearly inventory cost can be modeled mathematically.

In the Exercise Set of this section of your textbook, you will solve a rational equation to assist this store owner with this important financial question.

First Steps:

☐ **Take comprehensive notes** from your instructor's lecture and insert your notes into this section of the *Learning Guide*. Be sure to write down all examples, definitions, and other key concepts. Additional learning resources include the *Video Lecture Series*, the *PowerPoints*, and Section 7.6 of your textbook which begins on page 529.

☐ Complete the ***Concept and Vocabulary Check*** on page 536 of the textbook.

Guided Practice:

☐ Review each of the following ***Solved Problems*** and complete each ***Pencil Problem***.

Learning Objective #1: Solve rational equations.

✔ Solved Problem #1

1a. Solve: $\dfrac{x}{6} = \dfrac{1}{6} + \dfrac{x}{8}$

There are no restrictions on the variable because the variable does not appear in any denominator.

The LCD is 24.

$$\frac{x}{6} = \frac{1}{6} + \frac{x}{8}$$

$$24\left(\frac{x}{6}\right) = 24\left(\frac{1}{6} + \frac{x}{8}\right)$$

$$24 \cdot \frac{x}{6} = 24 \cdot \frac{1}{6} + 24 \cdot \frac{x}{8}$$

$$4x = 4 + 3x$$

$$x = 4$$

The solution set is $\{4\}$.

✎ Pencil Problem #1 ✎

1a. Solve: $\dfrac{4x}{3} = \dfrac{x}{18} - \dfrac{x}{6}$

Copyright © 2017 Pearson Education, Inc.

1b. Solve: $\dfrac{5}{2x} = \dfrac{17}{18} - \dfrac{1}{3x}$

The restriction is $x \neq 0$.

The LCD is $18x$.

$$\dfrac{5}{2x} = \dfrac{17}{18} - \dfrac{1}{3x}$$

$$18x\left(\dfrac{5}{2x}\right) = 18x\left(\dfrac{17}{18} - \dfrac{1}{3x}\right)$$

$$18x \cdot \dfrac{5}{2x} = 18x \cdot \dfrac{17}{18} - 18x \cdot \dfrac{1}{3x}$$

$$45 = 17x - 6$$

$$51 = 17x$$

$$3 = x$$

The solution set is $\{3\}$.

1b. Solve: $\dfrac{2}{x} + \dfrac{1}{3} = \dfrac{4}{x}$

1c. Solve: $x + \dfrac{6}{x} = -5$

The restriction is $x \neq 0$.

The LCD is x.

$$x + \dfrac{6}{x} = -5$$

$$x\left(x + \dfrac{6}{x}\right) = x(-5)$$

$$x \cdot x + x \cdot \dfrac{6}{x} = -5x$$

$$x^2 + 6 = -5x$$

$$x^2 + 5x + 6 = 0$$

$$(x+3)(x+2) = 0$$

$$x + 3 = 0 \quad \text{or} \quad x + 2 = 0$$

$$x = -3 \qquad\qquad x = -2$$

The solution set is $\{-3, -2\}$.

1c. Solve: $\dfrac{x}{5} - \dfrac{5}{x} = 0$

Copyright © 2017 Pearson Education, Inc.

1d. Solve: $\dfrac{x}{x-3} = \dfrac{3}{x-3} + 9$

The restriction is $x \neq 3$.

The LCD is $x - 3$.

$$\frac{x}{x-3} = \frac{3}{x-3} + 9$$

$$(x-3)\left(\frac{x}{x-3}\right) = (x-3)\left(\frac{3}{x-3} + 9\right)$$

$$\frac{x(x-3)}{x-3} = \frac{3(x-3)}{x-3} + 9(x-3)$$

$$x = 3 + 9(x-3)$$

$$x = 3 + 9x - 27$$

$$x = 9x - 24$$

$$-8x = -24$$

$$x = 3$$

The proposed solution, 3, is not a solution because of the restriction $x \neq 3$.

The solution set is $\{\ \}$.

1d. Solve: $\dfrac{8y}{y+1} = 4 - \dfrac{8}{y+1}$

Learning Objective #2: Solve problems involving formulas with rational expressions.	

✔ Solved Problem #2

2. The formula $y = \dfrac{250x}{100-x}$ models the cost, y, in millions of dollars, to remove x percent of a river's pollutants. If the government commits $750 million for this project, what percentage of pollutants can be removed?

$y = \dfrac{250x}{100-x}$

The restriction is $x \ne 100$.

$$750 = \dfrac{250x}{100-x}$$

$$(100-x)(750) = (100-x)\left(\dfrac{250x}{100-x}\right)$$

$$75,000 - 750x = 250x$$

$$75,000 = 1000x$$

$$75 = x$$

If government funding is increased to $750 million, then 75% of pollutants can be removed.

✎ Pencil Problem #2✎

2. In Palo Alto, California, a government agency ordered computer-related companies to contribute to a pool of money to clean up underground water supplies.

The formula $C = \dfrac{2x}{100-x}$ models the cost, C, in millions of dollars, for removing x percent of the contaminants. What percentage of the contaminants can be removed for $2 million?

Answers for Pencil Problems *(Textbook Exercise references in parentheses)*:

1a. $\{0\}$ *(7.6 #3)*   **1b.** $\{6\}$ *(7.6 #7)*   **1c.** $\{-5,5\}$ *(7.6 #19)*   **1d.** $\{\ \}$ *(7.6 #31)*

2. For $2 million, 50% of the contaminants can be removed. *(7.6 #57)*

Homework:

☐ **Review the Section 7.6 summary** on page 560 of the textbook.

☐ **Insert your homework** into this section of the *Learning Guide*. Show all work neatly and check your answers. Strive to work through difficulties when possible, making note of any exercises where you need additional help. Remember, even if your instructor assigns homework through *MyMathLab*, you should still write out your work.

   Copyright © 2017 Pearson Education, Inc.

Section 7.7
Applications Using Rational Equations and Proportions

What Does Your Footprint Reveal About You?

Height is proportional to foot length. In 1951, photos of large footprints were published. Some believed that these footprints were made by the "Abominable Snowman."

In the Exercise Set of the textbook, you will discover exactly how tall this "Abominable Snowman" was!

First Steps:

☐ **Take comprehensive notes** from your instructor's lecture and insert your notes into this section of the *Learning Guide*. Be sure to write down all examples, definitions, and other key concepts. Additional learning resources include the *Video Lecture Series*, the *PowerPoints*, and Section 7.7 of your textbook which begins on page 539.

☐ Complete the *Concept and Vocabulary Check* on page 548 of the textbook.

Guided Practice:

☐ Review each of the following *Solved Problems* and complete each *Pencil Problem*.

Learning Objective #1: Solve problems involving motion.

✔ *Solved Problem #1*	✎ *Pencil Problem #1* ✎

1. In still water, your average canoeing rate is 3 miles per hour. It takes you the same amount of time to travel 10 miles downstream, with the current, as 2 miles upstream, against the current. What is the rate of the water's current?

1. A jogger runs 4 miles per hour faster downhill than uphill. If the jogger can run 5 miles downhill in the same time that it takes to run 3 miles uphill, find the jogging rate in each direction.

Let x = the rate of the current.
Then $3 + x$ = the canoe's rate with the current.
and $3 - x$ = the canoe's rate against the current.

	Distance	Rate	Time $= \dfrac{\text{Distance}}{\text{Rate}}$
With the current	10	$3 + x$	$\dfrac{10}{3 + x}$
Against the current	2	$3 - x$	$\dfrac{2}{3 - x}$

Since the times are the same the equation is
$$\frac{10}{3 + x} = \frac{2}{3 - x}.$$

Use the cross-products principle to solve this equation.

$$\frac{10}{3+x} = \frac{2}{3-x}$$
$$10(3-x) = 2(3+x)$$
$$30 - 10x = 6 + 2x$$
$$30 - 12x = 6$$
$$-12x = -24$$
$$x = 2$$

The rate of the current is 2 miles per hour.

Learning Objective #2: Solve problems involving work.

✔ *Solved Problem #2*

2. One person can paint the outside of a house in 8 hours. A second person can do it in 4 hours. How long will it take them to do the job if they work together?

Let x = the number of hours for both people to paint a house together.

	Fractional part of job completed in 1 hour	Time working together	Fractional part of job completed in x hours
First person	$\dfrac{1}{8}$	x	$\dfrac{x}{8}$
Second person	$\dfrac{1}{4}$	x	$\dfrac{x}{4}$

Working together, the two people can complete the whole job, so $\dfrac{x}{8} + \dfrac{x}{4} = 1$.

Multiply both sides by the LCD, 8.

$$8\left(\frac{x}{8} + \frac{x}{4}\right) = 8 \cdot 1$$
$$x + 2x = 8$$
$$3x = 8$$
$$x = \frac{8}{3}$$
$$x = 2\frac{2}{3}$$

It will take $2\dfrac{2}{3}$ hours (or 2 hours 40 minutes) if they work together.

✎ *Pencil Problem #2* ✎

2. The water's current is 2 miles per hour. A boat can travel 6 miles downstream, with the current, in the same amount of time it travels 4 miles upstream, against the current. What is the boat's average rate in still water?

Copyright © 2017 Pearson Education, Inc.

Learning Objective #3: Solve problems involving proportions.

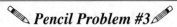

✔ *Solved Problem #3*	✎ *Pencil Problem #3*✎

3a. The property tax on a house with an assessed value of $250,000 is $3500. Determine the property tax on a house with an assessed value of $420,000, assuming the same tax rate.

3a. The tax on a property with an assessed value of $65,000 is $720. Find the tax on a property with an assessed value of $162,500.

Let $x =$ the property tax on the $420,000 house.

$$\frac{\text{Tax on \$250,000 house}}{\text{Assessed value (\$250,000)}} = \frac{\text{Tax on \$420,000 house}}{\text{Assessed value (\$420,000)}}$$

$$\frac{\$3500}{\$250,000} = \frac{\$x}{\$420,000}$$

$$\frac{3500}{250,000} = \frac{x}{420,000}$$

$$250,000x = (3500)(420,000)$$

$$250,000x = 1,470,000,000$$

$$\frac{250,000x}{250,000} = \frac{1,470,000,000}{250,000}$$

$$x = 5880$$

The property tax is $5880.

3b. Wildlife biologists catch, tag, and then release 120 deer back into a wildlife refuge. Two weeks later they observe a sample of 150 deer, 25 of which are tagged. Assuming the ratio of tagged deer in the sample holds for all deer in the refuge, approximately how many deer are in the refuge?

3b. St. Paul Island in Alaska has 12 fur seal rookeries (breeding places). In 1961, to estimate the fur seal pup population in the Gorbath rookery, 4963 fur seal pups were tagged in early August. In late August, a sample of 900 pups was observed and 218 of these were found to have been previously tagged. Estimate the total number of fur seal pups in this rookery.

Let $x =$ the total number of deer in the refuge.

$$\frac{120}{x} = \frac{25}{150}$$

$$25x = (120)(150)$$

$$25x = 18,000$$

$$\frac{25x}{25} = \frac{18,000}{25}$$

$$x = 720$$

There are about 720 deer in the refuge.

Copyright © 2017 Pearson Education, Inc.

Learning Objective #4: Solve problems involving similar triangles.

✔ *Solved Problem #4*

4. The similar triangles in the figure are shown with corresponding sides in the same relative position.

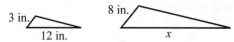

3 in.
8 in.
12 in.
x

Find the missing length, *x*.

$$\frac{3}{8} = \frac{12}{x}$$

$$3x = 8 \cdot 12$$

$$3x = 96$$

$$x = 32$$

The missing length is 32 inches.

✎ *Pencil Problem #4* ✎

4. The similar triangles in the figure are shown with corresponding sides in the same relative position.

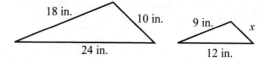

18 in.
10 in.
9 in.
x
24 in.
12 in.

Find the missing length, *x*.

Answers for Pencil Problems *(Textbook Exercise references in parentheses)*:

1. The jogger runs 10 miles per hour downhill and 6 miles per hour uphill. *(7.7 #3)*

2. 10 miles per hour. *(7.7 #9)*

3a. $1800 *(7.7 #17)*

3b. about 20,489 fur seal pups *(7.7 #19)*

4. 5 inches *(7.7 #25)*

Homework:

☐ **Review the Section 7.7 summary** which begins on page 560 of the textbook.

☐ **Insert your homework** into this section of the *Learning Guide*. Show all work neatly and check your answers. Strive to work through difficulties when possible, making note of any exercises where you need additional help. Remember, even if your instructor assigns homework through *MyMathLab*, you should still write out your work.

 Copyright © 2017 Pearson Education, Inc.

Section 7.8
Modeling Using Variation

How Far Would You Go To Lose Weight?

On the moon your weight would be significantly less.

To find out how much less, be sure to work on the application problems
in this section of your textbook!

First Steps:

☐ **Take comprehensive notes** from your instructor's lecture and insert your notes into this
section of the *Learning Guide*. Be sure to write down all examples, definitions, and other
key concepts. Additional learning resources include the *Video Lecture Series*, the
PowerPoints, and Section 7.8 of your textbook which begins on page 551.

☐ Complete the *Concept and Vocabulary Check* on page 555 of the textbook.

Guided Practice:

☐ Review each of the following *Solved Problems* and complete each *Pencil Problem*.

Learning Objective #1: Solve direct variation problems.

✔ *Solved Problem #1*

1. The number of gallons of water, W, used when
taking a shower varies directly as the time, t, in
minutes, in the shower. A shower lasting 5 minutes
uses 30 gallons of water. How much water is used in
a shower lasting 8 minutes?

Step 1 Write an equation. $W = kt$

Step 2 Use the given values to find k.
Substitute 30 for W and 5 for t.
$W = kt$
$30 = k \cdot 5$
$6 = k$

Step 3 Substitute the value of k into the equation
$W = 6t$

Step 4 Answer the problem's question. Substitute 8 for t
and solve for W.
$W = 6t$
$W = 6 \cdot 8$
$W = 48$

A shower lasting 8 minutes will use 48 gallons of water.

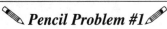 *Pencil Problem #1*

1. The cost, C, of an airplane ticket varies directly as
the number of miles, M, in the trip. A 3000-mile
trip costs \$400. What is the cost of a 450-mile trip?

Learning Objective #2: Solve inverse variation problems.

✔ Solved Problem #2

2. In general, if the temperature is constant, the pressure, P, of a gas in a container varies inversely as the volume, V, of the container. The pressure of a gas sample in a container whose volume is 8 cubic inches is 12 pounds per square inch. If the sample expands to a volume of 20 cubic inches, what is the new pressure of the gas?

Step 1 Write an equation. $P = \dfrac{k}{V}$

Step 2 Use the given values to find k.
Substitute 12 for P and 8 for V.

$$P = \frac{k}{V}$$

$$12 = \frac{k}{8}$$

$$12 \cdot 8 = k$$

$$96 = k$$

Step 3 Substitute the value of k into the equation.

$$P = \frac{96}{V}$$

Step 4 Answer the problem's question. Substitute 20 for V and solve for P.

$$P = \frac{96}{V}$$

$$P = \frac{96}{20}$$

$$P = 4.8$$

If the sample expands to a volume of 20 cubic inches, the new pressure of the gas will be 4.8 pounds per square inch.

✎ Pencil Problem #2 ✎

2. The volume of a gas in a container at a constant temperature varies inversely as the pressure. If the volume is 32 cubic centimeters at a pressure of 8 pounds per square centimeter, find the pressure when the volume is 40 cubic centimeters.

Answers for Pencil Problems *(Textbook Exercise references in parentheses)*:

1. $60 *(7.8 #15)*   **2.** 6.4 pounds per square centimeter *(7.8 #21)*

Homework:

☐ **Review the Section 7.8 summary** on page 562 of the textbook.

☐ **Insert your homework** into this section of the *Learning Guide*. Show all work neatly and check your answers. Strive to work through difficulties when possible, making note of any exercises where you need additional help. Remember, even if your instructor assigns homework through *MyMathLab*, you should still write out your work.

Copyright © 2017 Pearson Education, Inc.

Group members make up the sales team for a company that makes computer video games. It has been determined that the formula

$$y = \frac{200x}{x^2 + 100}$$

models the monthly sales, y, in thousands of games, of a new video game x months after the game is introduced.

The figure shows the graph of the formula.

Monthly Sales of a New Video Game

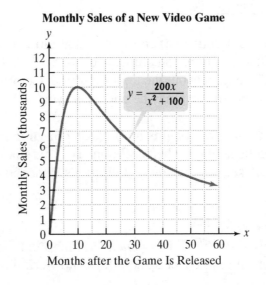

Months after the Game Is Released

a. What are the team's recommendations to the company in terms of how long the video game should be on the market before another new video game is introduced?

b. What other factors might members want to take into account in terms of the recommendations?

c. What will eventually happen to sales, and how is this indicated by the graph?

d. What could the company do to change the behavior of this model and continue generating sales? Would such changes be cost effective?

Getting Ready for the Chapter 7 Test

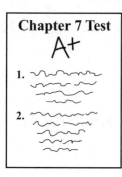

Chapter 7 Test

One of the best ways to prepare for a test is to stay on top of your studying, keeping up as your professor proceeds from section to section. Falling behind on one section often makes it difficult to understand the material in the following section. Never wait until the last minute to study for an exam.

Below are several actions that will help you stay organized as you prepare for your test.

How to prepare for your Chapter Test:

☐ **Write down any details that your instructor shares about the test.**
In addition to items such as location, date, time, and essentials to bring, be sure to listen carefully for specific information about the topics covered. Communicate with your instructor concerning any details that may be unclear to you.

☐ **Read the Chapter Summary that begins on page 557 of your textbook.**
Study the appropriate sections in the Chapter Summary. This summary contains the most important material in each section including, definitions, concepts, procedures, and examples.

☐ **Review your *Learning Guide*.**
Go back through the *Solved Problems* and *Pencil Problems* in this chapter of your *Learning Guide*. You may find it helpful to cover up solutions and work through the problems again.

☐ **Study your notes and homework.**
Read through your class notes that you took during this unit, and review the corresponding homework assignments.

☐ **Review quizzes and other feedback from your professor.**
Review any quizzes you have taken and be sure you understand any errors that you made. Seek help with any concepts that are still unclear.

☐ **Complete the Review Exercises that begin on page 562 of your textbook.**
Work the assigned problems from the Review Exercises. These exercises represent the most significant problems for each of the chapter's sections. The answers for all Review Exercises are in the back of your textbook.

☐ **Take the Chapter Test that begins on page 564 of your textbook.**
- Find a quiet place to take the Chapter Test.
- Do not use notes, index cards, or any resources other than those your instructor will allow during the actual test.
- After completing the entire test, check your answers in the back of the textbook.
- Watch the *Chapter Test Prep Video* to review any exercises you may have missed.

Copyright © 2017 Pearson Education, Inc.

Learning Objectives
1. Combine like terms.

Learning Objective #1: Combine like terms.

✔ *Solved Problem #1*	✎ *Pencil Problem #1*
1a. Combine like terms: $7x + 3x$	**1a.** Combine like terms: $7x + 10x$

$$7x + 3x = (7 + 3)x$$
$$= 10x$$

1b. Combine like terms: $9a - 4a$

$$9a - 4a = (9 - 4)a$$
$$= 5a$$

1b. Combine like terms: $11a - 3a$

1c. Simplify: $9x + 6y + 5x + 2y$

$$9x + 6y + 5x + 2y = 9x + 5x + 6y + 2y$$
$$= (9 + 5)x + (6 + 2)y$$
$$= 14x + 8y$$

1c. Simplify: $11a + 12 + 3a + 2$

Answers for Pencil Problems:

1a. $17x$ **1b.** $8a$ **1c.** $14a + 14$

Copyright © 2017 Pearson Education, Inc.

Section 8.1
Finding Roots

Be CAREFUL on the turns!!!

What is the maximum speed at which a racing cyclist can turn a corner
without tipping over?

The answer, in miles per hour, is given by an algebraic expression that involves
finding a square root.

In this section, we develop the basics of radical expressions,
and then apply them in various applications, including cycling.

First Steps:

☐ **Take comprehensive notes** from your instructor's lecture and insert your notes into this
section of the *Learning Guide*. Be sure to write down all examples, definitions, and other
key concepts. Additional learning resources include the *Video Lecture Series*, the
PowerPoints, and Section 8.1 of your textbook which begins on page 568.

☐ Complete the ***Concept and Vocabulary Check*** on page 574 of the textbook.

Guided Practice:

☐ Review each of the following ***Solved Problems*** and complete each ***Pencil Problem***.

Learning Objective #1: Find square roots.	
✔ *Solved Problem #1*	✎ *Pencil Problem #1* ✎
1a. Evaluate: $\sqrt{81}$	**1a.** Evaluate: $\sqrt{36}$
$\sqrt{81} = 9$ The principal square root of 81 is 9.	
1b. Evaluate: $\sqrt{\dfrac{1}{25}}$	**1b.** Evaluate: $\sqrt{\dfrac{1}{9}}$
$\sqrt{\dfrac{1}{25}} = \dfrac{1}{5}$ because $\left(\dfrac{1}{5}\right)^2 = \dfrac{1}{25}$.	
1c. Evaluate: $\sqrt{36+64}$	**1c.** Evaluate: $\sqrt{33-8}$
$\sqrt{36+64} = \sqrt{100} = 10$	

Copyright © 2017 Pearson Education, Inc.

1d. Evaluate: $\sqrt{36} + \sqrt{64}$

$$\sqrt{36} + \sqrt{64} = 6 + 8$$
$$= 14$$

1d. Evaluate: $\sqrt{144} + \sqrt{25}$

Learning Objective #2: Evaluate models containing square roots.

✔ Solved Problem #2

2. Racing cyclists use the formula $v = 4\sqrt{r}$ to determine the maximum velocity, v, in miles per hour, to turn a corner with radius r, in feet, without tipping over. Determine the maximum velocity that a cyclist should travel around a corner of radius 13 feet without tipping over.

$$v = 4\sqrt{r}$$
$$v = 4\sqrt{16}$$
$$v = 4 \cdot 4$$
$$v = 16$$

The maximum velocity that a cyclist should travel around a corner of radius 16 feet is 16 miles per hour.

✎ Pencil Problem #2 ✐

2. Racing cyclists use the formula $v = 4\sqrt{r}$ to determine the maximum velocity, v, in miles per hour, to turn a corner with radius r, in feet, without tipping over. What is the maximum velocity that a cyclist should travel around a corner of radius 4 feet without tipping over?

Learning Objective #3: Use a calculator to find decimal approximations for irrational square roots.

✔ Solved Problem #3

3. Use a calculator to approximate the expression. Round to two decimal places. $\sqrt{7}$

$$\sqrt{7} \approx 2.645751311 \approx 2.65$$

✎ Pencil Problem #3 ✐

3. Use a calculator to approximate the expression. Round to two decimal places. $\dfrac{-5 + \sqrt{321}}{6}$

Learning Objective #4: Use a calculator to evaluate models containing square roots.

✔ Solved Problem #3

4. The mathematical model $P = 2.2\sqrt{t} + 45$ describes the percentage of bachelor's degrees, P, awarded to women in U.S. colleges t years after 1975. Use the formula to find the percentage, to the nearest percent, of degrees awarded to women in 2005.

2005 is 30 years after 1975. Therefore, substitute 30 for t into the formula.

$$P = 2.2\sqrt{t} + 45$$
$$P = 2.2\sqrt{30} + 45 \approx 57$$

According to the model, about 57% of degrees were awarded to women in 2005.

✎ Pencil Problem #3 ✐

4. The mathematical model $y = 2.9\sqrt{x} + 36$ describes the head circumference of healthy children where y is the head circumference, in centimeters, at age x months, $0 \le x \le 14$. According to the model, what is the head circumference at 9 months?

Copyright © 2017 Pearson Education, Inc.

Learning Objective #5: Find higher roots.	
✔ *Solved Problem #4*	✎ *Pencil Problem #4* ✎
5a. Find the cube root: $\sqrt[3]{1}$	**5a.** Find the cube root: $\sqrt[3]{64}$
$\sqrt[3]{1} = 1$ because $1^3 = 1$.	
5b. Find the cube root: $\sqrt[3]{-27}$	**5b.** Find the cube root: $\sqrt[3]{-1000}$
$\sqrt[3]{-27} = -3$ because $(-3)^3 = -27$.	
5c. Find the cube root: $\sqrt[3]{\dfrac{1}{125}}$	**5c.** Find the cube root: $\sqrt[3]{\dfrac{1}{125}}$
$\sqrt[3]{\dfrac{1}{125}} = \dfrac{1}{5}$ because $\left(\dfrac{1}{5}\right)^3 = \dfrac{1}{125}$.	
5d. Find the indicated root: $\sqrt[4]{81}$	**5d.** Find the indicated root: $\sqrt[4]{16}$
$\sqrt[4]{81} = 3$ because $3^4 = 81$.	
5e. Find the indicated root: $\sqrt[4]{-81}$	**5e.** Find the indicated root: $\sqrt[4]{-16}$
$\sqrt[4]{-81}$ is not a real number because the index, 4, is even and the radicand, −81, is negative.	

Copyright © 2017 Pearson Education, Inc.

5f. Find the indicated root: $-\sqrt[4]{81}$

$-\sqrt[4]{81} = -3$ because $\sqrt[4]{81} = 3$.

5f. Find the indicated root: $-\sqrt[4]{256}$

5g. Find the indicated root: $\sqrt[5]{-\dfrac{1}{32}}$

$\sqrt[5]{-\dfrac{1}{32}} = -\dfrac{1}{2}$ because $\left(-\dfrac{1}{2}\right)^5 = -\dfrac{1}{32}$.

5g. Find the indicated root: $\sqrt[5]{-1}$

Answers for Pencil Problems *(Textbook Exercise references in parentheses)*:

1a. 6 *(8.1 #1)*   **1b.** $\dfrac{1}{3}$ *(8.1 #7)*   **1c.** 5 *(8.1 #17)*   **1d.** 17 *(8.1 #23)*

2. 8 miles per hour *(8.1 #85)*

3. 2.15 *(8.1 #41)*   **4.** 44.7cm *(8.1 #89b)*

5a. 4 *(8.1 #47)*   **5b.** −10 *(8.1 # 55)*   **5c.** $\dfrac{1}{5}$ *(8.1 # 53)*   **5d.** 2 *(8.1 #59)*

5e. not a real number *(8.1 #63)*   **5f.** −4 *(8.1 #69)*   **5g.** −1 *(8.1 #65)*

Homework:

☐ **Review the Section 8.1 summary** on page 617 of the textbook.

☐ **Insert your homework** into this section of the *Learning Guide*. Show all work neatly and check your answers. Strive to work through difficulties when possible, making note of any exercises where you need additional help. Remember, even if your instructor assigns homework through *MyMathLab*, you should still write out your work.

    Copyright © 2017 Pearson Education, Inc.

Section 8.2
Multiplying and Dividing Radicals

Radicals in Space???

What does travel in space have to do with radicals?

Imagine that in the future we will be able to travel at velocities approaching the speed of light (approximately 186,000 miles per second).

According to Einstein's theory of special relativity,
time would pass more quickly on Earth than it would in the moving spaceship.

First Steps:

☐ **Take comprehensive notes** from your instructor's lecture and insert your notes into this section of the *Learning Guide*. Be sure to write down all examples, definitions, and other key concepts. Additional learning resources include the *Video Lecture Series*, the *PowerPoints*, and Section 8.2 of your textbook which begins on page 578.

☐ Complete the *Concept and Vocabulary Check* on page 584 of the textbook.

Guided Practice:

☐ Review each of the following *Solved Problems* and complete each *Pencil Problem*.

Learning Objective #1: Multiply square roots.	
✔ *Solved Problem #1*	✎ *Pencil Problem #1* ✎
1a. Use the product rule for square roots to find the product: $\sqrt{3} \cdot \sqrt{10}$	**1a.** Use the product rule for square roots to find the product: $\sqrt{2} \cdot \sqrt{7}$
$\sqrt{3} \cdot \sqrt{10} = \sqrt{3 \cdot 10}$ $\qquad = \sqrt{30}$	
1b. Use the product rule for square roots to find the product: $\sqrt{2x} \cdot \sqrt{13y}$	**1b.** Use the product rule for square roots to find the product: $\sqrt{3x} \cdot \sqrt{5y}$
$\sqrt{2x} \cdot \sqrt{13y} = \sqrt{2x \cdot 13y}$ $\qquad = \sqrt{26xy}$	

1c. Use the product rule for square roots to find the product: $\sqrt{3} \cdot \sqrt{3}$

$$\sqrt{3} \cdot \sqrt{3} = \sqrt{9}$$
$$= 3$$

1c. Use the product rule for square roots to find the product: $\sqrt{5} \cdot \sqrt{5}$

Learning Objective #2: Simplify square roots.

✔ **Solved Problem #2**

2a. Simplify: $\sqrt{60}$

4 is the greatest perfect square that is a factor of 60.

$$\sqrt{60} = \sqrt{4 \cdot 15}$$
$$= \sqrt{4}\sqrt{15}$$
$$= 2\sqrt{15}$$

✐ **Pencil Problem #2** ✐

2a. Simplify: $\sqrt{50}$

2b. Simplify: $\sqrt{55}$

$\sqrt{55}$ cannot be simplified because it has no perfect square factors other than 1.

2b. Simplify: $\sqrt{35}$

2c. Simplify: $\sqrt{40x^{16}}$

$4x^{16}$ is the greatest perfect square that is a factor of $40x^{16}$.

$$\sqrt{40x^{16}} = \sqrt{4x^{16} \cdot 10}$$
$$= 2x^8\sqrt{10}$$

2c. Simplify: $\sqrt{20x^6}$

Copyright © 2017 Pearson Education, Inc.

2d. Multiply and then simplify: $\sqrt{15x^6} \cdot \sqrt{3x^7}$

$$\sqrt{15x^6} \cdot \sqrt{3x^7} = \sqrt{15x^6 \cdot 3x^7}$$
$$= \sqrt{45x^{13}}$$
$$= \sqrt{9x^{12} \cdot 5x}$$
$$= 3x^6\sqrt{5x}$$

2d. Multiply and then simplify: $\sqrt{15x^4} \cdot \sqrt{5x^9}$

Learning Objective #3: Use the quotient rule for square roots.

✔ **Solved Problem #3**

🖉 **Pencil Problem #3** 🖉

3a. Simplify: $\sqrt{\dfrac{49}{25}}$

$$\sqrt{\frac{49}{25}} = \frac{\sqrt{49}}{\sqrt{25}}$$
$$= \frac{7}{5}$$

3a. Simplify: $\sqrt{\dfrac{3}{4}}$

3b. Simplify: $\dfrac{\sqrt{48x^5}}{\sqrt{3x}}$

$$\frac{\sqrt{48x^5}}{\sqrt{3x}} = \sqrt{\frac{48x^5}{3x}}$$
$$= \sqrt{16x^4}$$
$$= 4x^2$$

3b. Simplify: $\dfrac{\sqrt{32x^3}}{\sqrt{8x}}$

Learning Objective #4: Use the product and quotient rules for other roots.

✔ **Solved Problem #4**

🖉 **Pencil Problem #4** 🖉

4a. Simplify: $\sqrt[3]{40}$

8 is the greatest perfect cube that is a factor of 40.

$$\sqrt[3]{40} = \sqrt[3]{8 \cdot 5}$$
$$= 2\sqrt[3]{5}$$

4a. Simplify: $\sqrt[3]{54}$

Copyright © 2017 Pearson Education, Inc.

4b. Simplify: $\sqrt[5]{8} \cdot \sqrt[5]{8}$

$$\sqrt[5]{8} \cdot \sqrt[5]{8} = \sqrt[5]{64}$$
$$= \sqrt[5]{32 \cdot 2}$$
$$= \sqrt[5]{32} \cdot \sqrt[5]{2}$$
$$= 2\sqrt[5]{2}$$

4b. Simplify: $\sqrt[4]{4} \cdot \sqrt[4]{8}$

4c. Simplify: $\sqrt[3]{\dfrac{125}{27}}$

$$\sqrt[3]{\frac{125}{27}} = \frac{\sqrt[3]{125}}{\sqrt[3]{27}}$$
$$= \frac{5}{3}$$

4c. Simplify: $\sqrt[3]{\dfrac{3}{8}}$

Answers for Pencil Problems *(Textbook Exercise references in parentheses)*:

1a. $\sqrt{14}$ *(8.2 #1)*   **1b.** $\sqrt{15xy}$ *(8.2 #3)*   **1c.** 5   *(8.2 #5)*

2a. $5\sqrt{2}$ *(8.2 #15)*   **2b.** $\sqrt{35}$ cannot be simplified   *(8.2 #25)*

2c. $2x^3\sqrt{5}$ *(8.2 #39)*   **2d.** $5x^6\sqrt{3x}$ *(8.2 #63)*

3a. $\dfrac{\sqrt{3}}{2}$ *(8.2 #71)*   **3b.** $2x$ *(8.2 #87)*

4a. $3\sqrt[3]{2}$ *(8.2 #95)*   **4b.** $2\sqrt[4]{2}$ *(8.2 #103)*   **4c.** $\dfrac{\sqrt[3]{3}}{2}$ *(8.2 #107)*

Homework:

☐ **Review the Section 8.2 summary** on page 617 of the textbook.

☐ **Insert your homework** into this section of the *Learning Guide*. Show all work neatly and check your answers. Strive to work through difficulties when possible, making note of any exercises where you need additional help. Remember, even if your instructor assigns homework through *MyMathLab*, you should still write out your work.

   Copyright © 2017 Pearson Education, Inc.

Section 8.3
Operations with Radicals

College and Jobs!!!!!!!

If you are a full-time college student with a job then you are part of the data for a radical model.

The mathematical model,
$$J = 1.4\sqrt{x} + 55 - (20 - 1.2\sqrt{x})$$
gives the percentage, J, of full-time college students with jobs x years after 1975.

In this section of your textbook, we will explore this function, and we will use the concepts of the section to simplify the formula to a manageable form.

First Steps:

☐ **Take comprehensive notes** from your instructor's lecture and insert your notes into this section of the *Learning Guide*. Be sure to write down all examples, definitions, and other key concepts. Additional learning resources include the *Video Lecture Series*, the *PowerPoints*, and Section 8.3 of your textbook which begins on page 587.

☐ Complete the *Concept and Vocabulary Check* on page 591 of the textbook.

Guided Practice:

☐ Review each of the following *Solved Problems* and complete each *Pencil Problem*.

Learning Objective #1: Add and subtract radicals.	
✔ *Solved Problem #1*	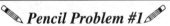 *Pencil Problem #1*
1a. Add or subtract as indicated: $8\sqrt{13} + 9\sqrt{13}$	**1a.** Add or subtract as indicated: $17\sqrt{6} - 2\sqrt{6}$

$$8\sqrt{13} + 9\sqrt{13} = (8+9)\sqrt{13}$$
$$= 17\sqrt{13}$$

1b. Add or subtract as indicated: $5\sqrt{27} + \sqrt{12}$

$$\begin{aligned}
5\sqrt{27} + \sqrt{12} &= 5\sqrt{9 \cdot 3} + \sqrt{4 \cdot 3} \\
&= 5 \cdot 3\sqrt{3} + 2\sqrt{3} \\
&= 15\sqrt{3} + 2\sqrt{3} \\
&= 17\sqrt{3}
\end{aligned}$$

1b. Add or subtract as indicated: $\sqrt{50} + \sqrt{18}$

1c. Add or subtract as indicated: $6\sqrt{18x} - 4\sqrt{8x}$

$$\begin{aligned}
6\sqrt{18x} - 4\sqrt{8x} &= 6\sqrt{9 \cdot 2x} - 4\sqrt{4 \cdot 2x} \\
&= 6 \cdot 3\sqrt{2x} - 4 \cdot 2\sqrt{2x} \\
&= 18\sqrt{2x} - 8\sqrt{2x} \\
&= 10\sqrt{2x}
\end{aligned}$$

1c. Add or subtract as indicated: $2\sqrt{45x} - 2\sqrt{20x}$

Learning Objective #2: Multiply radical expressions with more than one term.

✔ *Solved Problem #2*

✎ *Pencil Problem #2*✎

2a. Multiply: $\sqrt{2}\left(\sqrt{5} + \sqrt{11}\right)$

Use the distributive property.

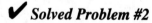

$$\begin{aligned}
\sqrt{2}\left(\sqrt{5} + \sqrt{11}\right) &= \sqrt{2}\sqrt{5} + \sqrt{2}\sqrt{11} \\
&= \sqrt{10} + \sqrt{22}
\end{aligned}$$

2a. Multiply: $\sqrt{7}\left(\sqrt{6} - \sqrt{10}\right)$

Copyright © 2017 Pearson Education, Inc.

2b. Multiply: $(4+\sqrt{3})(2+\sqrt{3})$

Use FOIL.

$$
\begin{aligned}
(4+\sqrt{3})(2+\sqrt{3}) &= 4 \cdot 2 + 4\sqrt{3} + 2\sqrt{3} + \left(\sqrt{3}\right)^2 \\
&= 8 + 4\sqrt{3} + 2\sqrt{3} + 3 \\
&= 11 + 6\sqrt{3}
\end{aligned}
$$

2b. Multiply: $(5+\sqrt{2})(6+\sqrt{2})$

2c. Multiply: $(3+\sqrt{5})(8-4\sqrt{5})$

Use FOIL.

$$
\begin{aligned}
(3+\sqrt{5})(8-4\sqrt{5}) &= 3 \cdot 8 - 3 \cdot 4\sqrt{5} + 8\sqrt{5} - 4\left(\sqrt{5}\right)^2 \\
&= 24 - 12\sqrt{5} + 8\sqrt{5} - 4 \cdot 5 \\
&= 24 - 12\sqrt{5} + 8\sqrt{5} - 20 \\
&= 4 - 4\sqrt{5}
\end{aligned}
$$

2c. Multiply: $(6-3\sqrt{7})(2-5\sqrt{7})$

Learning Objective #3: Multiply conjugates.

✔ *Solved Problem #3*

3a. Multiply: $(3+\sqrt{11})(3-\sqrt{11})$

Use the special-product formula
$(A+B)(A-B) = A^2 - B^2$.

$$
\begin{aligned}
(3+\sqrt{11})(3-\sqrt{11}) &= 3^2 - \left(\sqrt{11}\right)^2 \\
&= 9 - 11 \\
&= -2
\end{aligned}
$$

✎ *Pencil Problem #3* ✎

3a. Multiply: $(1-\sqrt{6})(1+\sqrt{6})$

3b. Multiply: $(\sqrt{7} - \sqrt{2})(\sqrt{7} + \sqrt{2})$

Use the special-product formula
$(A + B)(A - B) = A^2 - B^2$.

$$(\sqrt{7} - \sqrt{2})(\sqrt{7} + \sqrt{2}) = \left(\sqrt{7}\right)^2 - \left(\sqrt{2}\right)^2$$
$$= 7 - 2$$
$$= 5$$

3b. Multiply: $(2\sqrt{3} + 7)(2\sqrt{3} - 7)$

Answers for Pencil Problems *(Textbook Exercise references in parentheses)*:

1a. $15\sqrt{6}$ *(8.3 #3)*

1b. $8\sqrt{2}$ *(8.3 #27)*

1c. $2\sqrt{5x}$ *(8.3 #33)*

2a. $\sqrt{42} - \sqrt{70}$ *(8.3 #45)*

2b. $32 + 11\sqrt{2}$ *(8.3 #51)*

2c. $117 - 36\sqrt{7}$ *(8.3 #55)*

3a. -5 *(8.3 #65)*   **3b.** -37 *(8.3 #71)*

Homework:

☐ **Review the Section 8.3 summary** on page 618 of the textbook.

☐ **Insert your homework** into this section of the *Learning Guide*. Show all work neatly and check your answers. Strive to work through difficulties when possible, making note of any exercises where you need additional help. Remember, even if your instructor assigns homework through *MyMathLab*, you should still write out your work.

Copyright © 2017 Pearson Education, Inc.

Section 8.4
Rationalizing the Denominator

Are You Getting a Tax Refund?

In most tax years, approximately 59% of all taxpayers receive a tax refund, whereas 41% must pay more taxes than were withheld.

In this section's Exercise Set, you will use a formula that models the percentage of taxpayers who must pay more taxes based on the taxpayer's age. In the section itself, you will learn how to rewrite the formula without a radical in its denominator using a technique called rationalizing the denominator.

First Steps:

☐ **Take comprehensive notes** from your instructor's lecture and insert your notes into this section of the *Learning Guide*. Be sure to write down all examples, definitions, and other key concepts. Additional learning resources include the *Video Lecture Series*, the *PowerPoints*, and Section 8.4 of your textbook which begins on page 595.

☐ Complete the *Concept and Vocabulary Check* on page 599 of the textbook.

Guided Practice:

☐ Review each of the following *Solved Problems* and complete each *Pencil Problem*.

Learning Objective #1: Rationalize denominators containing one term.

✔ *Solved Problem #1*	✎ *Pencil Problem #1* ✎
1a. Rationalize the denominator: $\dfrac{25}{\sqrt{10}}$	**1a.** Rationalize the denominator: $\dfrac{2}{\sqrt{6}}$

Multiply the numerator and denominator by $\sqrt{10}$. Then simplify.

$$\frac{25}{\sqrt{10}} \cdot \frac{\sqrt{10}}{\sqrt{10}} = \frac{25\sqrt{10}}{10}$$

$$= \frac{5\sqrt{10}}{2}$$

1b. Rationalize the denominator: $\sqrt{\dfrac{2}{7}}$

The square root of a quotient is the quotient of the square roots.

$$\sqrt{\frac{2}{7}} = \frac{\sqrt{2}}{\sqrt{7}}$$

Multiply the numerator and denominator by $\sqrt{7}$ and then simplify.

$$\sqrt{\frac{2}{7}} = \frac{\sqrt{2}}{\sqrt{7}} \cdot \frac{\sqrt{7}}{\sqrt{7}}$$

$$= \frac{\sqrt{14}}{7}$$

1b. Rationalize the denominator: $\sqrt{\dfrac{3}{5}}$

1c. Rationalize the denominator: $\dfrac{15}{\sqrt{18}}$

Begin by simplifying $\sqrt{18}$.

$$\frac{15}{\sqrt{18}} = \frac{15}{3\sqrt{2}}$$

Multiply the numerator and denominator by $\sqrt{2}$ and then simplify.

$$\frac{15}{\sqrt{18}} = \frac{15}{3\sqrt{2}}$$

$$= \frac{15}{3\sqrt{2}} \cdot \frac{\sqrt{2}}{\sqrt{2}}$$

$$= \frac{15\sqrt{2}}{3 \cdot 2}$$

$$= \frac{5\sqrt{2}}{2}$$

1c. Rationalize the denominator: $\dfrac{1}{\sqrt{20}}$

Copyright © 2017 Pearson Education, Inc.

1d. Rationalize the denominator: $\sqrt{\dfrac{7x}{20}}$

The square root of a quotient is the quotient of the square roots.

$$\sqrt{\frac{7x}{20}} = \frac{\sqrt{7x}}{\sqrt{20}}$$

Next, simplify $\sqrt{20}$.

$$\sqrt{\frac{7x}{20}} = \frac{\sqrt{7x}}{\sqrt{20}}$$

$$= \frac{\sqrt{7x}}{2\sqrt{5}}$$

Multiply the numerator and denominator by $\sqrt{5}$ and then simplify.

$$\sqrt{\frac{7x}{20}} = \frac{\sqrt{7x}}{\sqrt{20}}$$

$$= \frac{\sqrt{7x}}{2\sqrt{5}} \cdot \frac{\sqrt{5}}{\sqrt{5}}$$

$$= \frac{\sqrt{35x}}{2 \cdot 5}$$

$$= \frac{\sqrt{35x}}{10}$$

1d. Rationalize the denominator: $\sqrt{\dfrac{x^2}{3}}$

Learning Objective #2: Rationalize denominators containing two terms.

✔ Solved Problem #2

2a. Rationalize the denominator: $\dfrac{8}{4+\sqrt{5}}$

Multiply the numerator and the denominator by the conjugate of the denominator.

$$\frac{8}{4+\sqrt{5}} = \frac{8}{4+\sqrt{5}} \cdot \frac{4-\sqrt{5}}{4-\sqrt{5}}$$

$$= \frac{32-8\sqrt{5}}{16-5}$$

$$= \frac{32-8\sqrt{5}}{11}$$

✎ Pencil Problem #2 ✎

2a. Rationalize the denominator: $\dfrac{1}{4+\sqrt{3}}$

2b. Rationalize the denominator: $\dfrac{8}{\sqrt{7}-\sqrt{3}}$

2b. Rationalize the denominator: $\dfrac{6}{\sqrt{6}+\sqrt{3}}$

Multiply the numerator and the denominator by the conjugate of the denominator.

$$\frac{8}{\sqrt{7}-\sqrt{3}} = \frac{8}{\sqrt{7}-\sqrt{3}} \cdot \frac{\sqrt{7}+\sqrt{3}}{\sqrt{7}+\sqrt{3}}$$

$$= \frac{8\sqrt{7}+8\sqrt{3}}{\left(\sqrt{7}\right)^2 - \left(\sqrt{3}\right)^2}$$

$$= \frac{8\sqrt{7}+8\sqrt{3}}{7-3}$$

$$= \frac{4\left(2\sqrt{7}+2\sqrt{3}\right)}{4}$$

$$= 2\sqrt{7}+2\sqrt{3}$$

<u>Answers</u> for Pencil Problems *(Textbook Exercise references in parentheses)*:

1a. $\dfrac{\sqrt{6}}{3}$ *(8.4 #5)*

1b. $\dfrac{\sqrt{15}}{5}$ *(8.4 #9)*

1c. $\dfrac{\sqrt{5}}{10}$ *(8.4 #25)*

1d. $\dfrac{x\sqrt{3}}{3}$ *(8.4 #13)*

2a. $\dfrac{4-\sqrt{3}}{13}$ *(8.4 #53)*

2b. $2\sqrt{6}-2\sqrt{3}$ *(8.4 #65)*

Homework:

☐ **Review the Section 8.4 summary** which begins on page 618 of the textbook.

☐ **Insert your homework** into this section of the *Learning Guide*. Show all work neatly and check your answers. Strive to work through difficulties when possible, making note of any exercises where you need additional help. Remember, even if your instructor assigns homework through *MyMathLab*, you should still write out your work.

Copyright © 2017 Pearson Education, Inc.

Section 8.5
Radical Equations

> ## How Much TV Do YOU Watch???
>
> Americans spend more of their free time watching TV than doing any other activity.
>
> In this section of the textbook, we will use a radical equation to explore the relationship between the average number of hours per week spent watching TV and annual income.

First Steps:

☐ **Take comprehensive notes** from your instructor's lecture and insert your notes into this section of the *Learning Guide*. Be sure to write down all examples, definitions, and other key concepts. Additional learning resources include the *Video Lecture Series*, the *PowerPoints*, and Section 8.5 of your textbook which begins on page 602.

☐ Complete the *Concept and Vocabulary Check* on page 607 of the textbook.

Guided Practice:

☐ Review each of the following *Solved Problems* and complete each *Pencil Problem*.

Learning Objective #1: Solve radical equations.	
✔ **Solved Problem #1**	✎ **Pencil Problem #1** ✎
1a. Solve: $\sqrt{2x+3} = 5$	**1a.** Solve: $\sqrt{x+2} = 3$

The radical is isolated; square both sides and solve the equation.

$$\sqrt{2x+3} = 5$$
$$\left(\sqrt{2x+3}\right)^2 = 5^2$$
$$2x+3 = 25$$
$$2x = 22$$
$$x = 11$$

Check 11:
$$\sqrt{2x+3} = 5$$
$$\sqrt{2 \cdot 11 + 3} = 5$$
$$\sqrt{25} = 5$$
$$5 = 5, \text{ true}$$

The true statement obtained from substituting 11 into the equation verifies that 11 is a solution.

The solution set is $\{11\}$.

1b. Solve: $\sqrt{x+32} - 3\sqrt{x} = 0$

First, isolate each radical.

$$\sqrt{x+32} - 3\sqrt{x} = 0$$
$$\sqrt{x+32} = 3\sqrt{x}$$

Square both sides, and then solve the equation.

$$\sqrt{x+32} = 3\sqrt{x}$$
$$\left(\sqrt{x+32}\right)^2 = \left(3\sqrt{x}\right)^2$$
$$x+32 = 9x$$
$$-8x = -32$$
$$x = 4$$

Check 4:

$$\sqrt{x+32} - 3\sqrt{x} = 0$$
$$\sqrt{4+32} - 3\sqrt{4} = 0$$
$$\sqrt{36} - 3\cdot 2 = 0$$
$$6 - 6 = 0$$
$$0 = 0, \text{ true}$$

The solution set is $\{4\}$.

1b. Solve: $3\sqrt{x-1} = \sqrt{3x+3}$

1c. Solve: $\sqrt{x} + 1 = 0$

First, isolate the radical.

$$\sqrt{x} + 1 = 0$$
$$\sqrt{x} = -1$$

Square both sides, and then solve the equation.

$$\sqrt{x} = -1$$
$$\left(\sqrt{x}\right)^2 = (-1)^2$$
$$x = 1$$

Check 1:

$$\sqrt{x} + 1 = 0$$
$$\sqrt{1} + 1 = 0$$
$$1 + 1 = 0$$
$$2 = 0, \text{ false}$$

The false statement indicates that 1 is not a solution.

The solution set is $\varnothing$.

1c. Solve: $3\sqrt{x} + 5 = 2$

Copyright © 2017 Pearson Education, Inc.

1d. Solve: $\sqrt{x+3}+3=x$

1d. Solve: $\sqrt{3x}+10=x+4$

First, isolate the radical.

$\sqrt{x+3}+3=x$

$\sqrt{x+3}=x-3$

Square both sides, and then solve the equation.

$\sqrt{x+3}=x-3$

$\left(\sqrt{x+3}\right)^2=(x-3)^2$

$x+3=x^2-6x+9$

$0=x^2-7x+6$

$0=(x-1)(x-6)$

$x-1=0$ or $x-6=0$

$x=1$ $x=6$

You must check both proposed solutions.

Check 1:   Check 6:

$\sqrt{x+3}+3=x$ $\sqrt{x+3}+3=x$

$\sqrt{1+3}+3=1$ $\sqrt{6+3}+3=6$

$\sqrt{4}+3=1$ $\sqrt{9}+3=6$

$2+3=1$ $3+3=6$

$5=1,$ false $6=6,$ true

The false statement obtained from substituting 1 into the equation indicates that 1 is not a solution.

The true statement obtained from substituting 6 into the equation indicates that 6 is a solution.

The solution set is $\{6\}$.

Learning Objective #2: Solve problems involving square-root models.

✔ *Solved Problem #2*	✎ *Pencil Problem #2*✎
2. The formula $H = -2.3\sqrt{I} + 67.6$ models weekly television viewing time, H, in hours, by annual income, I, in thousands of dollars. What annual income corresponds to 33.1 hours per week watching TV?	2. When firefighters are working to put out a fire, the rate at which they spray water on the fire depends on the nozzle pressure. The formula $f = 120\sqrt{p}$ models the water's flow rate, f, in gallons per minute, in terms of the nozzle pressure, p, in pounds per square inch. What nozzle pressure is needed to achieve a water flow rate of 840 gallons per minute?

$$H = -2.3\sqrt{I} + 67.6$$
$$33.1 = -2.3\sqrt{I} + 67.6$$
$$-34.5 = -2.3\sqrt{I}$$
$$\frac{-34.5}{-2.3} = \frac{-2.3\sqrt{I}}{-2.3}$$
$$15 = \sqrt{I}$$
$$15^2 = \left(\sqrt{I}\right)^2$$
$$225 = I$$

The model indicates that an annual income of 225 thousand dollars, or $225,000, corresponds to 33.1 hours per week watching TV.

Answers for Pencil Problems *(Textbook Exercise references in parentheses)*:

1a. {7} *(8.5 #5)*   **1b.** {2} *(8.5 #29)*   **1c.** ∅ , reject 1 *(8.5 # 43)*   **1d.** {12} , reject 3 *(8.5 #41)*

2. 49 pounds per square inch *(8.5 #55)*

Homework:

☐ **Review the Section 8.5 summary** on page 619 of the textbook.

☐ **Insert your homework** into this section of the *Learning Guide.* Show all work neatly and check your answers. Strive to work through difficulties when possible, making note of any exercises where you need additional help. Remember, even if your instructor assigns homework through *MyMathLab*, you should still write out your work.

 Copyright © 2017 Pearson Education, Inc.

Section 8.6
Rational Exponents

Go for a SPIN in Space!

To prevent bone and muscle loss for astronauts on lengthy space voyages, artificial gravity can be created in a space station. A rotating bedlike apparatus is used to create the artificial gravity.

The required rate of rotation is given by a formula that contains rational exponents. You will encounter this formula in the applications in the Exercise Set of your textbook.

First Steps:

☐ **Take comprehensive notes** from your instructor's lecture and insert your notes into this section of the *Learning Guide*. Be sure to write down all examples, definitions, and other key concepts. Additional learning resources include the *Video Lecture Series*, the *PowerPoints*, and Section 8.6 of your textbook which begins on page 610.

☐ Complete the *Concept and Vocabulary Check* on page 614 of the textbook.

Guided Practice:

☐ Review each of the following *Solved Problems* and complete each *Pencil Problem*.

Learning Objective #1: Evaluate expressions with rational exponents.	
✔ *Solved Problem #1*	✎ *Pencil Problem #1* ✎
1a. Simplify: $25^{\frac{1}{2}}$	**1a.** Simplify: $49^{\frac{1}{2}}$

The denominator of the exponent is the index of the radical. Thus an exponent of $\frac{1}{2}$ is equivalent to a square root.

$$25^{\frac{1}{2}} = \sqrt{25}$$
$$= 5$$

Copyright © 2017 Pearson Education, Inc.

1b. Simplify: $-81^{\frac{1}{4}}$

The denominator of the exponent is the index of the radical.

Note that the base is 81 and the negative sign is not affected by the exponent.

$$-81^{\frac{1}{4}} = -\sqrt[4]{81}$$
$$= -3$$

1b. Simplify: $-125^{\frac{1}{3}}$

1c. Simplify: $(-8)^{\frac{1}{3}}$

The denominator of the exponent is the index of the radical.

Note that the parentheses indicated that the base is -8. Thus the negative sign is affected by the exponent and should by under the radical.

$$(-8)^{\frac{1}{3}} = \sqrt[3]{-8}$$
$$= -2$$

1c. Simplify: $\left(\dfrac{27}{64}\right)^{\frac{1}{3}}$

1d. Simplify: $27^{\frac{4}{3}}$

The denominator, 3, is the radical's index and the numerator, 4, is the exponent.

$$27^{\frac{4}{3}} = \left(\sqrt[3]{27}\right)^4$$
$$= 3^4$$
$$= 81$$

1d. Simplify: $81^{\frac{3}{2}}$

Copyright © 2017 Pearson Education, Inc.

1e. Simplify: $4^{\frac{3}{2}}$

The denominator, 2, is the radical's index and the numerator, 3, is the exponent.

$$4^{\frac{3}{2}} = \left(\sqrt{4}\right)^3$$
$$= 2^3$$
$$= 8$$

1e. Simplify: $9^{\frac{3}{2}}$

1f. Simplify: $25^{-\frac{1}{2}}$

$$25^{-\frac{1}{2}} = \frac{1}{25^{\frac{1}{2}}}$$
$$= \frac{1}{\sqrt{25}}$$
$$= \frac{1}{5}$$

1f. Simplify: $9^{-\frac{1}{2}}$

1g. Simplify: $32^{-\frac{4}{5}}$

$$32^{-\frac{4}{5}} = \frac{1}{32^{\frac{4}{5}}}$$
$$= \frac{1}{\left(\sqrt[5]{32}\right)^4}$$
$$= \frac{1}{2^4}$$
$$= \frac{1}{16}$$

1g. Simplify: $81^{-\frac{5}{4}}$

Copyright © 2017 Pearson Education, Inc.

Learning Objective #2: Solve problems using models with rational exponents.	
✔ *Solved Problem #2*	✎ *Pencil Problem #2* ✎

2. The formula $W = 62x^{-\frac{7}{5}}$ models the percentage of women, W, who have never engaged in sexual activity with another person, where x is the group number designating the age ranges as follows:

Group 1	Group 2	Group 3
ages 15 - 17	ages 18 - 19	ages 20 - 24

2a. According to the formula, what percentage of women ages 20 – 24 have never engaged in sexual activity with another person? Use a calculator and round to the nearest percent.

Since this is group 3, substitute 3 for x.

$$W = 62x^{-\frac{7}{5}}$$

$$W = 62(3)^{-\frac{7}{5}} \approx 13$$

About 13% of women ages 20-24 have never engaged in sexual activity with another person.

2b. Rewrite the formula in radical notation.

$$W = 62x^{-\frac{7}{5}}$$

$$W = \frac{62}{x^{7/5}}$$

$$W = \frac{62}{\left(\sqrt[5]{x}\right)^7} \quad \text{or} \quad W = \frac{62}{\sqrt[5]{x^7}}$$

2. The formula $h = 0.84d^{\frac{2}{3}}$ models a tree's height, h, in meters, in terms of its base diameter, d, in centimeters.

2a. The largest known sequoia, the General Sherman in California, has a base diameter of 985 centimeters (about the size of a small house). Use a calculator to approximate the height of the General Sherman to the nearest tenth of a meter.

2b. Rewrite the formula in radical notation.

Answers for Pencil Problems (*Textbook Exercise references in parentheses*):

1a. 7 *(8.6 #1)* **1b.** −5 *(8.6 # 7)* **1c.** $\frac{3}{4}$ *(8.6 # 15)* **1d.** 729 *(8.6 #17)* **1e.** 27 *(8.6 #21)* **1f.** $\frac{1}{3}$ *(8.6 #25)*

1g. $\frac{1}{243}$ *(8.6 #35)* **2a.** 83.2 meters *(8.6 #57a)* **2b.** $h = 0.84\left(\sqrt[3]{d}\right)^2$ or $h = 0.84\sqrt[3]{d^2}$ *(8.6 #57b)*

Homework:

☐ **Review the Section 8.6 summary** on page 619 of the textbook.

☐ **Insert your homework** into this section of the *Learning Guide*. Show all work neatly and check your answers. Strive to work through difficulties when possible, making note of any exercises where you need additional help. Remember, even if your instructor assigns homework through *MyMathLab*, you should still write out your work.

  Copyright © 2017 Pearson Education, Inc.

Group Project for Chapter 8

The following topics related to irrational roots are appropriate for a group research project. A group report should be given to the class on the researched topic.

a. A History of How Irrational Numbers Developed

b. Proving that $\sqrt{2}$ Is Irrational

c. Golden Rectangles in Art and Architecture
(See Exercise Set 8.4, Exercise 85 on page 601 of the textbook.)

d. Golden Ratios in Proportions of the Human Body
(See Exercise Set 8.4, Exercise 85 on page 601 of the textbook.)

e. Radicals in Nature

Getting Ready for the Chapter 8 Test

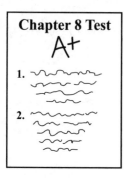

Chapter 8 Test

One of the best ways to prepare for a test is to stay on top of your studying, keeping up as your professor proceeds from section to section. Falling behind on one section often makes it difficult to understand the material in the following section. Never wait until the last minute to study for an exam.

Below are several actions that will help you stay organized as you prepare for your test.

How to prepare for your Chapter Test:

☐ **Write down any details that your instructor shares about the test.**
In addition to items such as location, date, time, and essentials to bring, be sure to listen carefully for specific information about the topics covered. Communicate with your instructor concerning any details that may be unclear to you.

☐ **Read the Chapter Summary that begins on page 617 of your textbook.**
Study the appropriate sections in the Chapter Summary. This summary contains the most important material in each section including, definitions, concepts, procedures, and examples.

☐ **Review your *Learning Guide.***
Go back through the *Solved Problems* and *Pencil Problems* in this chapter of your *Learning Guide.* You may find it helpful to cover up solutions and work through the problems again.

☐ **Study your notes and homework.**
Read through your class notes that you took during this unit, and review the corresponding homework assignments.

☐ **Review quizzes and other feedback from your professor.**
Review any quizzes you have taken and be sure you understand any errors that you made. Seek help with any concepts that are still unclear.

☐ **Complete the Review Exercises that begin on page 619 of your textbook.**
Work the assigned problems from the Review Exercises. These exercises represent the most significant problems for each of the chapter's sections. The answers for all Review Exercises are in the back of your textbook.

☐ **Take the Chapter Test on page 621 of your textbook.**
  • Find a quiet place to take the Chapter Test.
  • Do not use notes, index cards, or any resources other than those your instructor will allow during the actual test.
  • After completing the entire test, check your answers in the back of the textbook.
  • Watch the *Chapter Test Prep Video* to review any exercises you may have missed.

Copyright © 2017 Pearson Education, Inc.

Chapter 9.R Quadratic Equations and Introduction to Functions
Integrated Review

Learning Objectives
1. Use point plotting to graph linear equations.
2. Solve quadratic equations by factoring.

Learning Objective #1: Use point plotting to graph linear equations.

✔ *Solved Problem #1*

1a. Graph the equation: $y = 2x$

First, make a table of values:

x	$y = 2x$	(x, y)
−2	$y = 2(-2) = -4$	$(-2, -4)$
−1	$y = 2(-1) = -2$	$(-1, -2)$
0	$y = 2(0) = 0$	$(0, 0)$
1	$y = 2(1) = 2$	$(1, 2)$
2	$y = 2(2) = 4$	$(2, 4)$

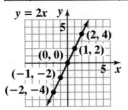

✎ *Pencil Problem #1* ✎

1a. Graph the equation: $y = x$

1b. Graph the equation: $y = \frac{1}{2}x + 2$

First, make a table of values:

x	$y = \frac{1}{2}x + 2$	(x, y)
−4	$y = \frac{1}{2}(-4) + 2 = 0$	$(-4, 0)$
−2	$y = \frac{1}{2}(-2) + 2 = 1$	$(-2, 1)$
0	$y = \frac{1}{2}(0) + 2 = 2$	$(0, 2)$
2	$y = \frac{1}{2}(2) + 2 = 3$	$(2, 3)$
4	$y = \frac{1}{2}(4) + 2 = 4$	$(4, 4)$

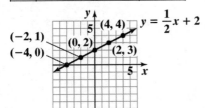

1b. Graph the equation: $y = -\frac{3}{2}x + 1$

Learning Objective #2: Solve quadratic equations by factoring.

✔ **Solved Problem #2**	✎ **Pencil Problem #2** ✎

2a. Solve: $x^2 - 6x + 5 = 0$

All the terms are on one side and zero is on the other side.

$x^2 - 6x + 5 = 0$

Thus, factor the left side of the equation.

$x^2 - 6x + 5 = 0$

$(x-1)(x-5) = 0$

Next, set each factor equal to zero and solve the resulting equations.

$x - 1 = 0$ or $x - 5 = 0$

$x = 1$ $x = 5$

The solution set is $\{1, 5\}$.

2a. Solve: $x^2 - 5x = 0$

2b. Solve: $4x^2 = 2x$

Move all terms to one side and obtain zero on the other side.

$4x^2 = 2x$

$4x^2 - 2x = 0$

Then factor the left side of the equation.

$4x^2 - 2x = 0$

$2x(2x - 1) = 0$

Next, set each factor equal to zero and solve the resulting equations.

$2x = 0$ or $2x - 1 = 0$

$x = 0$ $2x = 1$

$x = \dfrac{1}{2}$

The solution set is $\left\{0, \dfrac{1}{2}\right\}$.

2b. Solve: $2x^2 = 7x + 4$

Copyright © 2017 Pearson Education, Inc.

2c. Solve: $x^2 = 10x - 25$

Move all terms to one side and obtain zero on the other side.

$$x^2 = 10x - 25$$
$$x^2 - 10x + 25 = 0$$

Then factor the left side of the equation.

$$x^2 - 10x + 25 = 0$$
$$(x-5)^2 = 0$$

Because both factors are the same, it is only necessary to set one of them equal to zero.

$$x - 5 = 0$$
$$x = 5$$

The solution set is $\{5\}$.

2d. Solve: $(x-5)(x-2) = 28$

Write the equation in standard form by finding the product on the left side and then subtracting 28 from both sides.

$$(x-5)(x-2) = 28$$
$$x^2 - 7x + 10 = 28$$
$$x^2 - 7x - 18 = 0$$

Then factor the left side of the equation.

$$x^2 - 7x - 18 = 0$$
$$(x-9)(x+2) = 0$$

Set each factor equal to zero and solve the resulting equations.

$$x^2 - 7x - 18 = 0$$
$$(x-9)(x+2) = 0$$
$$x - 9 = 0 \quad \text{or} \quad x + 2 = 0$$
$$x = 9 \qquad\qquad x = -2$$

The solution set is $\{-2, 9\}$.

2c. Solve: $x^2 + 4x + 4 = 0$

2d. Solve: $x(x-4) = 21$

Copyright © 2017 Pearson Education, Inc.

Answers for Pencil Problems:

1a.

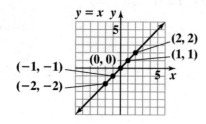

1b. $y = -\dfrac{3}{2}x + 1$

2a. $\{0,5\}$ **2b.** $\left\{-\dfrac{1}{2}, 4\right\}$ **2c.** $\{-2\}$ **2d.** $\{-3,7\}$

  Copyright © 2017 Pearson Education, Inc.

Section 9.1
Solving Quadratic Equations by the Square Root Property

Making a Splash!!!!!!!

In this section of the textbook, we will look at how a quadratic function can be used to model the distance an object will fall over a particular amount of time, such as a rock being dropped off a cliff into the water below.

First Steps:

☐ **Take comprehensive notes** from your instructor's lecture and insert your notes into this section of the *Learning Guide*. Be sure to write down all examples, definitions, and other key concepts. Additional learning resources include the *Video Lecture Series*, the *PowerPoints*, and Section 9.1 of your textbook which begins on page 624.

☐ Complete the *Concept and Vocabulary Check* on page 631 of the textbook.

Guided Practice:

☐ Review each of the following *Solved Problems* and complete each *Pencil Problem*.

Learning Objective #1: Solve quadratic equations using the square root property.	
✔ *Solved Problem #1*	✎ *Pencil Problem #1✎*
1a. Solve by the square root property: $x^2 = 36$	**1a.** Solve by the square root property: $y^2 = 81$
$x^2 = 36$ $x = \sqrt{36}$ or $x = -\sqrt{36}$ $x = 6 \qquad x = -6$ The solution set is $\{\pm 6\}$.	
1b. Solve by the square root property: $5x^2 = 15$	**1b.** Solve by the square root property: $4y^2 = 49$
$5x^2 = 15$ $\dfrac{5x^2}{5} = \dfrac{15}{5}$ $x^2 = 3$ $x = \sqrt{3}$ or $x = -\sqrt{3}$ The solution set is $\{\pm\sqrt{3}\}$.	

1c. Solve by the square root property: $2x^2 - 7 = 0$

$2x^2 - 7 = 0$

$\quad 2x^2 = 7$

$\quad\quad x^2 = \dfrac{7}{2}$

$x = \sqrt{\dfrac{7}{2}} \ \text{ or } \ x = -\sqrt{\dfrac{7}{2}}$

$x = \pm\sqrt{\dfrac{7}{2}}$

$\quad = \pm\dfrac{\sqrt{7}}{\sqrt{2}}\cdot\dfrac{\sqrt{2}}{\sqrt{2}}$

$\quad = \pm\dfrac{\sqrt{14}}{2}$

The solution set is $\left\{\pm\dfrac{\sqrt{14}}{2}\right\}$.

1c. Solve by the square root property: $2x^2 + 1 = 51$

1d. Solve by the square root property: $(x-3)^2 = 25$

$(x-3)^2 = 25$

$x - 3 = \sqrt{25} \ \text{ or } \ x - 3 = -\sqrt{25}$

$x - 3 = 5 \quad\ \text{ or } \ x - 3 = -5$

$\quad x = 8 \quad\quad\quad\quad x = -2$

The solution set is $\{-2, 8\}$.

1d. Solve by the square root property: $(x+5)^2 = 121$

1e. Solve by the square root property: $(x-2)^2 = 7$

$(x-2)^2 = 7$

$x - 2 = \sqrt{7} \quad\ \text{ or } \quad x - 2 = -\sqrt{7}$

$\quad x = 2 + \sqrt{7} \quad\quad\quad x = 2 - \sqrt{7}$

The solution set is $\left\{2 \pm \sqrt{7}\right\}$.

1e. Solve by the square root property: $(x-5)^2 = 3$

·Copyright © 2017 Pearson Education, Inc.

Learning Objective #2: Solve problems using the Pythagorean Theorem.

✔ **Solved Problem #2**

2. The dimensions of an old TV screen are 19.2 inches by 25.6 inches. What is the size of the screen?

$$19.2^2 + 25.6^2 = c^2$$
$$368.64 + 655.36 = c^2$$
$$1024 = c^2$$

$$c = \sqrt{1024} \quad \text{or} \quad c = -\sqrt{1024}$$
$$c = 32 \qquad\qquad c = -32$$

The dimension must be positive. Reject –32.
The size of the screen is 32 inches.

✎ **Pencil Problem #2** ✎

2. A square flower bed is to be enlarged by adding 2 meters on each side. If the larger square has an area of 144 square meters, what is the length of the original square?

Learning Objective #3: Find the distance between two points.	
✔ *Solved Problem #3*	✎ *Pencil Problem #3*✎
3. Find the distance between $(-4, 9)$ and $(1, -3)$.	**3.** Find the distance between $(-4, 2)$ and $(4, 17)$.

$$d = \sqrt{(x_2 - x_1)^2 + (y_2 - y_1)^2}$$
$$= \sqrt{(1 - (-4))^2 + (-3 - 9)^2}$$
$$= \sqrt{(5)^2 + (-12)^2}$$
$$= \sqrt{25 + 144}$$
$$= \sqrt{169}$$
$$= 13$$

The distance between the two points is 13 units.

Answers for Pencil Problems *(Textbook Exercise references in parentheses)*:

1a. $\{\pm 9\}$ *(9.1 #3)*

1b. $\left\{\pm\dfrac{7}{2}\right\}$ *(9.1 #11)*

1c. $\{\pm 5\}$ *(9.1 #13)*

1d. $\{-16, 6\}$ *(9.1 #21)*

1e. $\left\{5 \pm \sqrt{3}\right\}$ *(9.1 #25)*

2. 8 meters *(9.1 #79)*

3. 17 units *(9.1 #51)*

Homework:

☐ **Review the Section 9.1 summary** on page 679 of the textbook.

☐ **Insert your homework** into this section of the *Learning Guide.* Show all work neatly and check your answers. Strive to work through difficulties when possible, making note of any exercises where you need additional help. Remember, even if your instructor assigns homework through *MyMathLab*, you should still write out your work.

  Copyright © 2017 Pearson Education, Inc.

Section 9.2
Solving Quadratic Equations by Completing the Square

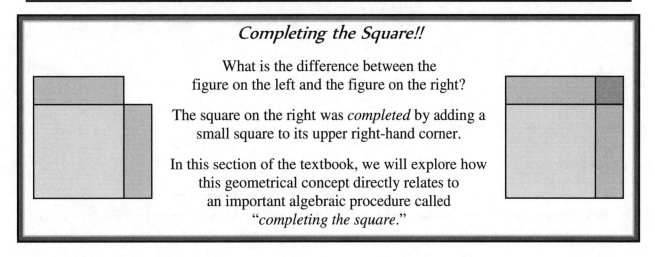

Completing the Square!!

What is the difference between the
figure on the left and the figure on the right?

The square on the right was *completed* by adding a
small square to its upper right-hand corner.

In this section of the textbook, we will explore how
this geometrical concept directly relates to
an important algebraic procedure called
"completing the square."

First Steps:

☐ **Take comprehensive notes** from your instructor's lecture and insert your notes into this
section of the *Learning Guide*. Be sure to write down all examples, definitions, and other
key concepts. Additional learning resources include the *Video Lecture Series*, the
PowerPoints, and Section 9.2 of your textbook which begins on page 634.

☐ Complete the *Concept and Vocabulary Check* on page 638 of the textbook.

Guided Practice:

☐ Review each of the following *Solved Problems* and complete each *Pencil Problem*.

Learning Objective #1: Complete the square of a binomial.

✔ *Solved Problem #1*	✏ *Pencil Problem #1*
1a. Complete the square for the binomial. Then factor the resulting trinomial: $x^2 + 10x$	**1a.** Complete the square for the binomial. Then factor the resulting trinomial: $x^2 + 10x$

$x^2 + 10x$

The coefficient of the *x*-term is 10. Half of 10 is 5, and
$5^2 = 25$. Add 25.

$$x^2 + 10x + 25 = (x + 5)^2$$

1b. Complete the square for the binomial. Then factor the resulting trinomial: $x^2 - 6x$

$x^2 - 6x$

The coefficient of the x-term is -6.

Half of -6 is -3, and $(-3)^2 = 9$. Add 9.

$x^2 - 6x + 9 = (x - 3)^2$

1b. Complete the square for the binomial. Then factor the resulting trinomial: $x^2 - 2x$

1c. Complete the square for the binomial. Then factor the resulting trinomial: $x^2 + 3x$

$x^2 + 3x$

The coefficient of the x-term is 3.

Half of 3 is $\dfrac{3}{2}$, and $\left(\dfrac{3}{2}\right)^2 = \dfrac{9}{4}$. Add $\dfrac{9}{4}$.

$x^2 + 3x + \dfrac{9}{4} = \left(x + \dfrac{3}{2}\right)^2$

1c. Complete the square for the binomial. Then factor the resulting trinomial: $x^2 - 7x$

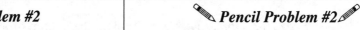

Learning Objective #2: Solve quadratic equations by completing the square.

✔ Solved Problem #2

✎ Pencil Problem #2 ✎

2a. Solve by completing the square: $x^2 + 6x = 7$

The coefficient of the x-term is 6. Half of 6 is 3, and $3^2 = 9$. Add 9 to both sides of the equation.

$x^2 + 6x = 7$

$x^2 + 6x + 9 = 7 + 9$

Factor, and then solve using the square root property.

$x^2 + 6x + 9 = 7 + 9$

$(x + 3)^2 = 16$

$x + 3 = \sqrt{16}$ or $x + 3 = -\sqrt{16}$

$x + 3 = 4$ $\qquad x + 3 = -4$

$x = 1$ $\qquad\quad x = -7$

The solution set is $\{-7, 1\}$.

2a. Solve by completing the square: $x^2 - 10x = -24$

Copyright © 2017 Pearson Education, Inc.

2b. Solve by completing the square: $x^2 - 10x + 18 = 0$

First subtract 18 from both sides to isolate the binomial.

$x^2 - 10x + 18 = 0$

$x^2 - 10x \quad = -18$

Next, complete the square by adding $\left(\dfrac{-10}{2}\right)^2$ to both sides.

$x^2 - 10x + 25 = -18 + 25$

$x^2 - 10x + 25 = 7$

Factor, and then solve using the square root property.

$x^2 - 10x + 25 = 7$

$(x - 5)^2 = 7$

$\begin{array}{lll} x - 5 = \sqrt{7} & \text{or} & x - 5 = -\sqrt{7} \\ \quad x = 5 + \sqrt{7} & & \quad x = 5 - \sqrt{7} \end{array}$

The solution set is $\left\{ 5 \pm \sqrt{7} \right\}$.

2b. Solve by completing the square: $x^2 + 4x + 1 = 0$

2c. Solve by completing the square: $2x^2 - 10x - 1 = 0$

$2x^2 - 10x - 1 = 0$

First, divide both sides of the equation by 2 so that the coefficient of the x^2 term will be 1.

$\dfrac{2x^2}{2} - \dfrac{10x}{2} - \dfrac{1}{2} = \dfrac{0}{2}$

$x^2 - 5x - \dfrac{1}{2} = 0$

Next, add $\dfrac{1}{2}$ to both sides to isolate the binomial.

$x^2 - 5x - \dfrac{1}{2} = 0$

$x^2 - 5x \quad = \dfrac{1}{2}$

(continued on next page)

2c. Solve by completing the square: $2x^2 - 2x - 6 = 0$

Copyright © 2017 Pearson Education, Inc.

Complete the square:

The coefficient of the x-term is -5, and $\frac{1}{2}(-5) = -\frac{5}{2}$, so

add $\left(-\frac{5}{2}\right)^2 = \frac{25}{4}$ to both sides.

$x^2 - 5x \qquad = \frac{1}{2}$

$x^2 - 5x + \frac{25}{4} = \frac{1}{2} + \frac{25}{4}$

$x^2 - 5x + \frac{25}{4} = \frac{2}{4} + \frac{25}{4}$

$\left(x - \frac{5}{2}\right)^2 = \frac{27}{4}$

$x - \frac{5}{2} = \sqrt{\frac{27}{4}}$ \qquad or \qquad $x - \frac{5}{2} = -\sqrt{\frac{27}{4}}$

$x = \frac{5}{2} + \frac{\sqrt{27}}{2}$ \qquad\qquad $x = \frac{5}{2} - \frac{\sqrt{27}}{2}$

$x = \frac{5}{2} + \frac{3\sqrt{3}}{2}$ \qquad\qquad $x = \frac{5}{2} - \frac{3\sqrt{3}}{2}$

$x = \frac{5 + 3\sqrt{3}}{2}$ \qquad\qquad $x = \frac{5 - 3\sqrt{3}}{2}$

The solution set is $\left\{\frac{5 \pm 3\sqrt{3}}{2}\right\}$.

Answers for Pencil Problems *(Textbook Exercise references in parentheses)*:

1a. $x^2 + 10x + 25 = (x+5)^2$ *(9.2 #1)* **1b.** $x^2 - 2x + 1 = (x-1)^2$ *(9.2 #3)*

1c. $x^2 - 7x + \frac{49}{4} = \left(x - \frac{7}{2}\right)^2$ *(9.2 #7)*

2a. $\{4,6\}$ *(9.2 #15)* **2b.** $\{-2 \pm \sqrt{3}\}$ *(9.2 #19)* **2c.** $\left\{\frac{1 \pm \sqrt{13}}{2}\right\}$ *(9.2 #27)*

Homework:

☐ **Review the Section 9.2 summary** that begins on page 679 of the textbook.

☐ **Insert your homework** into this section of the *Learning Guide*. Show all work neatly and check your answers. Strive to work through difficulties when possible, making note of any exercises where you need additional help. Remember, even if your instructor assigns homework through *MyMathLab*, you should still write out your work.

 Copyright © 2017 Pearson Education, Inc.

Section 9.3
The Quadratic Formula

Math and Today's News!

It may come as a surprise that mathematics, including quadratic equations, can be used to help us understand and explain many of the trends we experience in our lives.

The bar graph below shows undocumented immigrants living in the United States as a percentage of the foreign-born population.

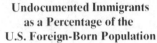

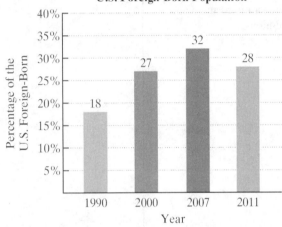

Source: Pew Hispanic Center

This data can also be modeled by a mathematical model.

This mathematical model is the following quadratic: $p = -0.05x^2 + 1.5x + 18$ where p is the percentage of the U.S. foreign-born who were undocumented immigrants x years after 1990.

In this section of your textbook will explore this quadratic model to explore where this trend is heading.

First Steps:

☐ **Take comprehensive notes** from your instructor's lecture and insert your notes into this section of the *Learning Guide*. Be sure to write down all examples, definitions, and other key concepts. Additional learning resources include the *Video Lecture Series*, the *PowerPoints*, and Section 9.3 of your textbook which begins on page 640.

☐ Complete the ***Concept and Vocabulary Check*** on page 647 of the textbook.

Guided Practice:

☐ Review each of the following **Solved Problems** and complete each **Pencil Problem**.

Learning Objective #1: Solve quadratic equations using the quadratic formula.

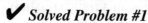 **Solved Problem #1**

1a. Solve using the quadratic formula:
$$8x^2 + 2x - 1 = 0$$

Identify the values of a, b, and c:
$a = 8$, $b = 2$, and $c = -1$.

Substitute these values into the quadratic formula and simplify to get the equation's solutions.

$$x = \frac{-b \pm \sqrt{b^2 - 4ac}}{2a}$$

$$x = \frac{-2 \pm \sqrt{2^2 - 4(8)(-1)}}{2(8)}$$

$$= \frac{-2 \pm \sqrt{4 + 32}}{16}$$

$$= \frac{-2 \pm \sqrt{36}}{16}$$

$$= \frac{-2 \pm 6}{16}$$

$$x = \frac{-2 + 6}{16} \quad \text{or} \quad x = \frac{-2 - 6}{16}$$

$$= \frac{4}{16} = \frac{1}{4} \qquad\qquad = \frac{-8}{16} = -\frac{1}{2}$$

The solution set is $\left\{ -\frac{1}{2}, \frac{1}{4} \right\}$.

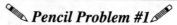 **Pencil Problem #1**

1a. Solve using the quadratic formula:
$$6x^2 - 5x - 6 = 0$$

Copyright © 2017 Pearson Education, Inc.

1b. Solve using the quadratic formula: $x^2 = 6x - 4$

Write the equation in standard form.
$$x^2 = 6x - 4$$

$$x^2 - 6x + 4 = 0$$

Identify the values of a, b, and c:
$a = 1$, $b = -6$, and $c = 4$.

Substitute these values into the quadratic formula and simplify to get the equation's solutions.

$$x = \frac{-b \pm \sqrt{b^2 - 4ac}}{2a}$$

$$x = \frac{-(-6) \pm \sqrt{(-6)^2 - 4(1)(4)}}{2(1)}$$

$$= \frac{6 \pm \sqrt{36 - 16}}{2}$$

$$= \frac{6 \pm \sqrt{20}}{2}$$

$$= \frac{6 \pm 2\sqrt{5}}{2}$$

$$= 3 \pm \sqrt{5}$$

The solution set is $\left\{ 3 \pm \sqrt{5} \right\}$.

1b. Solve using the quadratic formula: $x^2 - x = 14$

Learning Objective #2:
Determine the most efficient method to use when solving a quadratic equation.

✔ Solved Problem #2

2. What is the most efficient method for solving a quadratic equation of the form $ax^2 + c = 0$?

The most efficient method is to solve for x^2 and apply the square root property.

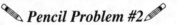 Pencil Problem #2

2. What is the most efficient method for solving a quadratic equation of the form $u^2 = d$, where u is a first-degree polynomial?

Copyright © 2017 Pearson Education, Inc.

Learning Objective #3: Solve problems using quadratic equations.

✔ Solved Problem #3

3. The percentage, p, of the United States population that was foreign-born x years after 1920 can be modeled by the formula $p = 0.004x^2 - 0.35x + 13.9$. According to this model, in which year will 25% of the United States population be foreign-born?

$p = 0.004x^2 - 0.35x + 13.9$

$25 = 0.004x^2 - 0.35x + 13.9$

$0 = 0.004x^2 - 0.35x - 11.1$

Identify the values of $a, b,$ and c:

$a = 0.004, b = -0.35,$ and $c = -11.1$.

Substitute these values into the quadratic formula and simplify to get the equation's solutions.

$x = \dfrac{-b \pm \sqrt{b^2 - 4ac}}{2a}$

$x = \dfrac{-(-0.35) \pm \sqrt{(-0.35)^2 - 4(0.004)(-11.1)}}{2(0.004)}$

$\approx -25 \text{ or } 112$

Reject the negative solution to the quadratic equation because the time cannot be negative. 25% of the United States population will be foreign-born 112 years after 1920, or 2032.

✎ Pencil Problem #3 ✎

3. A football is kicked straight up from a height of 4 feet with an initial speed of 60 feet per second.

The formula $h = -16t^2 + 60t + 4$ describes the ball's height above the ground, h, in feet, t seconds after it is kicked. How long will it take for the football to hit the ground? Use a calculator and round to the nearest tenth of a second.

Answers for Pencil Problems *(Textbook Exercise references in parentheses)*:

1a. $\left\{ -\dfrac{2}{3}, \dfrac{3}{2} \right\}$ *(9.3 #11)*   **1b.** $\left\{ \dfrac{1 \pm \sqrt{57}}{2} \right\}$ *(9.3 # 15)*

2. Use the square root property.   *(9.3 #43)*   **3.** about 3.8 seconds   *(9.3 #53)*

Homework:

☐ **Review the Section 9.3 summary** on page 680 of the textbook.

☐ **Insert your homework** into this section of the *Learning Guide*. Show all work neatly and check your answers. Strive to work through difficulties when possible, making note of any exercises where you need additional help. Remember, even if your instructor assigns homework through *MyMathLab*, you should still write out your work.

 Copyright © 2017 Pearson Education, Inc.

Section 9.4
Imaginary Numbers as Solutions of Quadratic Equations

Why Study Something if it is *IMAGINARY*???

Great Question!
The numbers that we study in this section were given the name "*imaginary*" at a time when mathematicians believed such numbers to be useless.

Since that time, many *real-life* applications for so-called imaginary numbers have been discovered, but the name they were originally given has endured.

First Steps:

☐ **Take comprehensive notes** from your instructor's lecture and insert your notes into this section of the *Learning Guide*. Be sure to write down all examples, definitions, and other key concepts. Additional learning resources include the *Video Lecture Series*, the *PowerPoints*, and Section 9.4 of your textbook which begins on page 651.

☐ Complete the *Concept and Vocabulary Check* on page 654 of the textbook.

Guided Practice:

☐ Review each of the following *Solved Problems* and complete each *Pencil Problem*.

Learning Objective #1: Express square roots of negative numbers in terms of i.

✔ *Solved Problem #1*	✎ *Pencil Problem #1* ✎
1a. Write as a multiple of i: $\sqrt{-16}$	**1a.** Write as a multiple of i: $\sqrt{-36}$
$\begin{aligned} \sqrt{-16} &= \sqrt{16(-1)} \\ &= \sqrt{16}\sqrt{-1} \\ &= 4i \end{aligned}$	
1b. Write as a multiple of i: $\sqrt{-50}$	**1b.** Write as a multiple of i: $\sqrt{-20}$
$\begin{aligned} \sqrt{-50} &= \sqrt{50(-1)} \\ &= \sqrt{25 \cdot 2}\sqrt{-1} \\ &= 5i\sqrt{2} \end{aligned}$	

Copyright © 2017 Pearson Education, Inc.

Learning Objective #2: Solve quadratic equations with imaginary solutions.

✔ **Solved Problem #2**	✏ *Pencil Problem #2* ✏
2a. Solve: $(x+2)^2 = -25$	**2a.** Solve: $(x+7)^2 = -64$

Use the square root property.

$$x + 2 = \sqrt{-25} \quad \text{or} \quad x + 2 = -\sqrt{-25}$$
$$x + 2 = 5i \qquad\qquad x + 2 = -5i$$
$$x = -2 + 5i \qquad\qquad x = -2 - 5i$$

The solution set is $\{-2 \pm 5i\}$.

2b. Solve: $x^2 + 6x + 13 = 0$

Use the quadratic formula with $a = 1$, $b = 6$, and $c = 13$.

$$x = \frac{-b \pm \sqrt{b^2 - 4ac}}{2a}$$
$$= \frac{-6 \pm \sqrt{6^2 - 4(1)(13)}}{2 \cdot 1}$$
$$= \frac{-6 \pm \sqrt{-16}}{2}$$
$$= \frac{-6 \pm 4i}{2}$$
$$= -3 \pm 2i$$

The solution set is $\{-3 \pm 2i\}$.

2b. Solve: $x^2 - 12x + 40 = 0$

Answers for Pencil Problems *(Textbook Exercise references in parentheses)*:

1a. $6i$ *(9.4 #1)*   **1b.** $2i\sqrt{5}$ *(9.4 #7)*   **2a.** $\{-7 \pm 8i\}$ *(9.4 #19)*   **2b.** $\{6 \pm 2i\}$ *(9.4 #29)*

Homework:

☐ **Review the Section 9.4 summary** that begins on page 680 of the textbook.

☐ **Insert your homework** into this section of the *Learning Guide*. Show all work neatly and check your answers. Strive to work through difficulties when possible, making note of any exercises where you need additional help. Remember, even if your instructor assigns homework through *MyMathLab*, you should still write out your work.

 Copyright © 2017 Pearson Education, Inc.

Section 9.5
Graphs of Quadratic Equations

Heads UP!!!

Many sports involve objects that are thrown, kicked, or hit,
and then proceed with no additional force of their own.
Such objects are called projectiles.

In this section of your textbook, you will learn to use graphs of quadratic equations to
gain a visual understanding of various projectile sports.

First Steps:

☐ **Take comprehensive notes** from your instructor's lecture and insert your notes into this section of the *Learning Guide*. Be sure to write down all examples, definitions, and other key concepts. Additional learning resources include the *Video Lecture Series*, the *PowerPoints*, and Section 9.5 of your textbook which begins on page 656.

☐ Complete the *Concept and Vocabulary Check* on page 665 of the textbook.

Guided Practice:

☐ Review each of the following *Solved Problems* and complete each *Pencil Problem*.

Learning Objective #1: Understand the characteristics of graphs of quadratic equations.	
✔ *Solved Problem #1*	✐ *Pencil Problem #1* ✐
1. Determine whether the graph of $y = x^2 - 6x + 8$ is a parabola that opens upward or downward.	1. Determine whether the graph of $y = -2x^2 + x + 6$ is a parabola that opens upward or downward.
Because a, the coefficient of x^2, is 1, which is greater than 0, the parabola opens upward.	

Learning Objective #2: Find a parabola's intercepts.	
✔ *Solved Problem #2*	✐ *Pencil Problem #2* ✐
2a. Find the x-intercepts for the parabola whose equation is $y = x^2 - 6x + 8$.	2a. Find the x-intercepts for the parabola whose equation is $y = x^2 - 4x + 3$.

Replace y with 0 and solve the resulting equation.

$0 = x^2 - 6x + 8$

$0 = (x - 4)(x - 2)$

$x - 4 = 0$ or $x - 2 = 0$

$x = 4$ $\qquad$ $x = 2$

The x-intercepts are 2 and 4.

2b. Find the *y*-intercept for the parabola whose equation is $y = x^2 - 6x + 8$.

To find the *y*-intercept, replace *x* with 0.

$y = x^2 - 6x + 8$

$y = 0^2 - 6(0) + 8$

$\quad = 8$

The *y*-intercept is 8.

2b. Find the *y*-intercept for the parabola whose equation is $y = -x^2 + 8x - 12$.

Learning Objective #3: Find a parabola's vertex.

✔ **Solved Problem #3**

3. Find the vertex for the parabola whose equation is $y = x^2 - 6x + 8$.

Note that $a = 1$, $b = -6$, $c = 8$.

x-coordinate of vertex: $x = \dfrac{-b}{2a} = \dfrac{-(-6)}{2(1)} = \dfrac{6}{2} = 3$

y-coordinate of vertex: $y = x^2 - 6x + 8$

$\qquad\qquad y = 3^2 - 6(3) + 8$

$\qquad\qquad\quad = 9 - 18 + 8$

$\qquad\qquad\quad = -1$

The vertex is (3, –1).

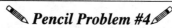 **Pencil Problem #3**

3. Find the vertex for the parabola whose equation is $y = 2x^2 + 4x - 6$.

Learning Objective #4: Graph quadratic equations.

✔ **Solved Problem #4**

4. Graph the quadratic equation: $y = x^2 + 6x + 5$

Step 1 Determine how the parabola opens.

Here *a*, the coefficient of x^2, is 1.

Because $a > 0$, the parabola opens upward.

Step 2 Find the vertex.

For this equation, $a = 1, b = 6$, and $c = 5$.

x-coordinate of vertex: $x = \dfrac{-b}{2a} = \dfrac{-6}{2(1)} = \dfrac{-6}{2} = -3$

y-coordinate of vertex: $y = x^2 + 6x + 5$

$\qquad\qquad\qquad y = (-3)^2 + 6(-3) + 5 = -4$

The vertex is $(-3, -4)$.

Pencil Problem #4

4. Graph the quadratic equation: $y = -x^2 + 4x - 3$

Copyright © 2017 Pearson Education, Inc.

Step 3 Find the *x*-intercepts.

Replace *y* with 0 in $y = x^2 + 6x + 5$ and solve for *x*.

$$x^2 + 6x + 5 = 0$$
$$(x+5)(x+1) = 0$$
$$x+5 = 0 \quad \text{or} \quad x+1 = 0$$
$$x = -5 \qquad x = -1$$

The *x*-intercepts are −5 and −1.

Step 4 Find the *y*-intercept.
Replace *x* with 0 and solve for *y*.

$$y = 0^2 + 6(0) + 5 = 5$$

The *y*-intercept is 5.

Steps 5 and 6 Plot the intercepts and the vertex.
Plot $(-3,-4), (-5,0), (-1,0),$ and $(0,5),$ and connect them with a smooth curve.

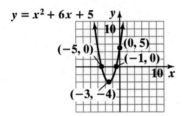

Learning Objective #5: Solve problems using a parabola's vertex.

✔ Solved Problem #5

5. An archer's arrow follows a parabolic path. The height of the arrow, *y*, in feet, can be modeled by $y = -0.005x^2 + 2x + 5$, where *x* is the arrow's horizontal distance, in feet.

5a. What is the maximum height of the arrow and how far from its release does this occur?

The information needed is found at the vertex.
x-coordinate of vertex:

$$x = \frac{-b}{2a} = \frac{-2}{2(-0.005)} = 200$$

y-coordinate of vertex:

$$y = -0.005x^2 + 2x + 5$$
$$y = -0.005(200)^2 + 2(200) + 5 = 205$$

The vertex is (200,205).

The maximum height of the arrow is 205 feet.
This occurs 200 feet from its release.

✏ Pencil Problem #5 ✏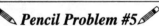

5. A ball is thrown upward and outward from a height of 6 feet. The height of the ball, *y*, in feet, can be modeled by $y = -0.8x^2 + 3.2x + 6$ where *x* is the ball's horizontal distance, in feet, from where it was thrown.

5a. What is the maximum height of the ball and how far from where it was thrown does this occur?

5b. Find the horizontal distance the arrow travels before it hits the ground. Round to the nearest foot.

5b. How far does the ball travel horizontally before hitting the ground?
Round to the nearest tenth of a foot.

The arrow will hit the ground when the height reaches 0.

$$y = -0.005x^2 + 2x + 5$$

$$0 = -0.005x^2 + 2x + 5$$

$$x = \frac{-b \pm \sqrt{b^2 - 4ac}}{2a}$$

$$x = \frac{-2 \pm \sqrt{2^2 - 4(-0.005)(5)}}{2(-0.005)}$$

$$x \approx -2 \ \text{ or } \ x \approx 402$$

The arrow travels 402 feet before hitting the ground.

Answers for Pencil Problems *(Textbook Exercise references in parentheses)*:

1. downward   *(9.5 #3)*

2a. 1 and 3   *(9.5 #5)*   **2b.** −12   *(9.5 #13)*

3. $(-1, -8)$ *(9.5 #21)*

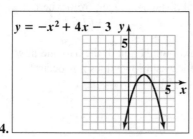

4.   *(9.5 #29)*

5a. The maximum height is 9.2 feet; this occurs 2 feet from its release.   *(9.5 #49a)*   **5b.** 5.4 feet   *(9.5 #49b)*

Homework:

☐ **Review the Section 9.5 summary** on page 681 of the textbook.

☐ **Insert your homework** into this section of the *Learning Guide*. Show all work neatly and check your answers. Strive to work through difficulties when possible, making note of any exercises where you need additional help. Remember, even if your instructor assigns homework through *MyMathLab*, you should still write out your work.

   Copyright © 2017 Pearson Education, Inc.

Section 9.6
Introduction to Functions

Say *WHAT*???

Along the way in this textbook, you have noticed that mathematical notation occasionally can have more than one meaning depending on the context.

For example, $(-3, 6)$ could refer to the ordered pair where $x = -3$ and $y = 6$, or it could refer to the open interval $-3 < x < 6$.

Similarly, in this section of the textbook, we will use the notation, $f(x)$. It may surprise you to find out that it does *not* mean to multiply "f times x."

It will be important for you to gain an understanding of what this notation *does* mean as you work through this essential concept of "functions."

$$f(x) \qquad f(x) \qquad f(x)$$

First Steps:

☐ **Take comprehensive notes** from your instructor's lecture and insert your notes into this section of the *Learning Guide*. Be sure to write down all examples, definitions, and other key concepts. Additional learning resources include the *Video Lecture Series*, the *PowerPoints*, and Section 9.6 of your textbook which begins on page 668.

☐ Complete the *Concept and Vocabulary Check* on page 675 of the textbook.

Guided Practice:

☐ Review each of the following *Solved Problems* and complete each *Pencil Problem*.

Learning Objective #1: Find the domain and range of a relation.

✔ *Solved Problem #1*

1. The following set shows calories burned per hour in various activities.
   Find the domain and range of the relation:
   {(golf, 250), (lawn mowing, 325),
   (water skiing, 430), (hiking, 430), (bicycling, 720)}.

The domain is the set of all first components.

Domain:
{golf, lawn mowing, water skiing, hiking, bicycling}

The range is the set of all second components.

Range:
{250, 325, 430, 720}

✎ *Pencil Problem #1*✎

1. Find the domain and range of the relation:
   {(1, 2), (3, 4), (5, 5)}

Copyright © 2017 Pearson Education, Inc.

Learning Objective #2: Determine whether a relation is a function.

✔ *Solved Problem #2*	✎ *Pencil Problem #2* ✎
2a. Determine whether the relation is a function: $$\{(1,2),(3,4),(6,5),(8,5)\}$$ Every element in the domain corresponds to exactly one element in the range. No two ordered pairs in the given relation have the same first component and different second components. Thus, the relation is a function.	**2a.** Determine whether the relation is a function: $$\{(-3,-3),(-2,-2),(-1,-1),(0,0)\}$$
2b. Determine whether the relation is a function: $$\{(1,2),(3,4),(5,6),(5,8)\}$$ 5 corresponds to both 6 and 8. If any element in the domain corresponds to more than one element in the range, the relation is not a function. Thus, the relation is not a function.	**2b.** Determine whether the relation is a function: $$\{(1,4),(1,5),(1,6)\}$$

Learning Objective #3: Evaluate a function.

✔ *Solved Problem #3*	✎ *Pencil Problem #3* ✎
3a. If $f(x)=4x+3$, find $f(5)$, $f(-2)$, and $f(0)$. $f(x)=4x+3$ $f(5)=4(5)+3$ $\quad=20+3$ $\quad=23$ $f(x)=4x+3$ $f(-2)=4(-2)+3$ $\quad=-8+3$ $\quad=-5$ $f(x)=4x+3$ $f(0)=4(0)+3$ $\quad=0+3$ $\quad=3$	**3a.** If $f(x)=8x-3$, find $f(12)$, $f\left(-\dfrac{1}{2}\right)$, and $f(0)$.

Copyright © 2017 Pearson Education, Inc.

3b. If $g(x) = x^2 + 4x + 3$,

find $g(5)$, $g(-4)$, and $g(0)$.

$g(x) = x^2 + 4x + 3$

$g(5) = (5)^2 + 4(5) + 3$

$\quad = 25 + 20 + 3$

$\quad = 48$

$g(x) = x^2 + 4x + 3$

$g(-4) = (-4)^2 + 4(-4) + 3$

$\quad = 16 - 16 + 3$

$\quad = 3$

$g(x) = x^2 + 4x + 3$

$g(0) = 0^2 + 4(0) + 3$

$\quad = 0 + 0 + 3$

$\quad = 3$

3b. If $g(x) = x^2 + 3x$,

find $g(2)$, $g(-2)$, and $g(0)$.

Learning Objective #4: Use the vertical line test to identify functions.

✔ *Solved Problem #4*

4. Use the vertical line test to determine if the graph represents y as a function of x.

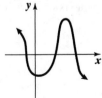

The graph passes the vertical line test and thus y is a function of x.

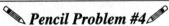 *Pencil Problem #4*

4. Use the vertical line test to determine if the graph represents y as a function of x.

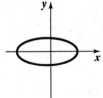

Copyright © 2017 Pearson Education, Inc.

Learning Objective #5: Find function values for functions that model data.

✔ **Solved Problem #5**	✏ **Pencil Problem #5** ✏
5. The linear function $f(x) = 0.5x + 65$ and the quadratic function $g(x) = -0.005x^2 + 0.67x + 64$ model the percentage of college freshman x years after 1980 who considered being well-off financially essential or very important. Which model serves as a better description for the freshman class of 2000?	**5.** The function $p(x) = 0.08x^2 - 1.8x + 42$ models the percentage of college freshman, $p(x)$, who studied and did homework at least six hours per week as high school seniors x years after 1992. Find and interpret $p(20)$.

$f(x) = 0.5x + 65$

$f(20) = 0.5(20) + 65 = 75$

According to the linear function, 75% of college freshman considered being well-off financially essential or very important in 2000.

$g(x) = -0.005x^2 + 0.67x + 64$

$g(20) = -0.005(20)^2 + 0.67(20) + 64 = 75.4$

According to the quadratic function, 75.4% of college freshman considered being well-off financially essential or very important in 2000.

According to the bar graph, 74% of college freshman considered being well-off financially essential or very important in 2000. Thus the linear function serves as a better description of this data.

Answers for Pencil Problems *(Textbook Exercise references in parentheses)*:

1. Domain: $\{1,3,5\}$; Range: $\{2,4,5\}$ *(9.6 #1)*

2a. function   *(9.6 #5)*   **2b.** not a function   *(9.6 #7)*

3a. $f(12) = 93$; $f\left(-\dfrac{1}{2}\right) = -7$; $f(0) = -3$ *(9.6 #13)*   **3b.** $g(2) = 10$; $g(-2) = -2$; $g(0) = 0$ *(9.6 #15)*

4. y is not a function of x *(9.6 #29)*

5. $p(20) = 38$; In 2012, or 20 years after 1992, 38% of college freshman had spent six or more hours per week studying during their high school senior year.   *(9.6 #45)*

Homework:

☐ **Review the Section 9.6 summary** on page 682 of the textbook.

☐ **Insert your homework** into this section of the *Learning Guide*. Show all work neatly and check your answers. Strive to work through difficulties when possible, making note of any exercises where you need additional help. Remember, even if your instructor assigns homework through *MyMathLab*, you should still write out your work.

   Copyright © 2017 Pearson Education, Inc.

Group Project for Chapter 9

The bar graph on page 677 of the textbook that is associated with Exercises 41 and 42 of Exercise Set 9.6 illustrates that if a relation is a function, reversing the components in each of its ordered pairs may result in a relation that is no longer a function.

Group members should find examples of bar graphs that illustrate this idea. Consult almanacs, newspapers, magazines, or the Internet. The group should select the graph with the most intriguing data.

For the graph selected, write and solve a problem with four parts similar to Exercise 41 or 42 as given here:

a. Write a set of five ordered pairs which correspond to the data selected.

b. Is the relation in part (a) a function? Explain your answer.

c. Again, write a set of five ordered pairs which correspond to the data selected, but this time reverse the way you write the points by interchanging the domain and range.

d. Is the relation in part (c) a function?

Copyright © 2017 Pearson Education, Inc.

Getting Ready for the Chapter 9 Test

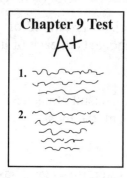

One of the best ways to prepare for a test is to stay on top of your studying, keeping up as your professor proceeds from section to section. Falling behind on one section often makes it difficult to understand the material in the following section. Never wait until the last minute to study for an exam.

Below are several actions that will help you stay organized as you prepare for your test.

How to prepare for your Chapter Test:

☐ **Write down any details that your instructor shares about the test.**
In addition to items such as location, date, time, and essentials to bring, be sure to listen carefully for specific information about the topics covered. Communicate with your instructor concerning any details that may be unclear to you.

☐ **Read the Chapter Summary that begins on page 679 of your textbook.**
Study the appropriate sections in the Chapter Summary. This summary contains the most important material in each section including, definitions, concepts, procedures, and examples.

☐ **Review your *Learning Guide.***
Go back through the *Solved Problems* and *Pencil Problems* in this chapter of your *Learning Guide*. You may find it helpful to cover up solutions and work through the problems again.

☐ **Study your notes and homework.**
Read through your class notes that you took during this unit, and review the corresponding homework assignments.

☐ **Review quizzes and other feedback from your professor.**
Review any quizzes you have taken and be sure you understand any errors that you made. Seek help with any concepts that are still unclear.

☐ **Complete the Review Exercises that begin on page 682 of your textbook.**
Work the assigned problems from the Review Exercises. These exercises represent the most significant problems for each of the chapter's sections. The answers for all Review Exercises are in the back of your textbook.

☐ **Take the Chapter Test that begins on page 684 of your textbook.**
- Find a quiet place to take the Chapter Test.
- Do not use notes, index cards, or any resources other than those your instructor will allow during the actual test.
- After completing the entire test, check your answers in the back of the textbook.
- Watch the *Chapter Test Prep Video* to review any exercises you may have missed.

Copyright © 2017 Pearson Education, Inc.

Appendix
Mean, Median, and Mode

What's the Hardest Thing to Do In COLLEGE?

It would be difficult to give a definitive answer to that question. But for many students, it often seems impossible to calculate a grade-point average (GPA).

One common system for finding GPA:

A = 4
B = 3
C = 2
D = 1
F = 0

Each course grade is weighted according to the number of credits of the course, thus, GPA is called a weighted mean.

In the Exercise Set for this appendix, you will apply the techniques of this section to calculate the GPA for the Grade Report shown below.

Grade Report		
GPA: ?????		
Course	**Credits**	**Grade**
Sociology	3	A
Biology	3.5	C
Music	1	B
Math	4	B
English	3	C

First Steps:

☐ **Take comprehensive notes** from your instructor's lecture and insert your notes into this section of the *Learning Guide*. Be sure to write down all examples, definitions, and other key concepts. Additional learning resources include the *Video Lecture Series*, the *PowerPoints*, and the Appendix of your textbook which begins on page 687.

Guided Practice:

☐ Review each of the following *Solved Problems* and complete each *Pencil Problem*.

Copyright © 2017 Pearson Education, Inc.

Learning Objective #1: Determine the mean of a set of data items.

✔ *Solved Problem #1*	✎ *Pencil Problem #1*

1. Find the mean earnings, in millions of dollars, for the following earnings, given in millions of dollars:

$$\$13, \$13, \$10, \$10, \$10, \$9, \$9, \$7, \$7, \$7$$

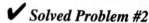

$$\text{Mean} = \frac{\sum x}{n}$$
$$= \frac{13+13+10+10+10+9+9+7+7+7}{10}$$
$$= \frac{95}{10}$$
$$= 9.5$$

The mean earning is $9.5 million

1. Find the mean for the following data:
$$91, 95, 99, 97, 93, 95$$

Learning Objective #2: Determine the median of a set of data items.

✔ *Solved Problem #2*	✎ *Pencil Problem #2*

2a. Find the median for the following data:
$$28, 42, 40, 25, 35$$

First arrange the data items from smallest to largest:

25, 28, <u>35</u>, 40, 42

The number of data items is odd, so the median is the middle number.

The median is 35.

2a. Find the median for the following data:
$$100, 40, 70, 40, 60$$

Copyright © 2017 Pearson Education, Inc.

2b. Find the median for the following data:
72, 61, 85, 93, 79, 87

First arrange the data items from smallest to largest:

61, 72, <u>79</u>, <u>85</u>, 87, 93

The number of data items is even, so the median is the mean of the two middle data items.

The median is $\dfrac{79+85}{2} = \dfrac{164}{2} = 82$.

2b. Find the median for the following data:
7, 4, 3, 2, 8, 5, 1, 3

Learning Objective #3: Determine the mode of a set of data items.

✔ Solved Problem #3

3a. Find the mode for the following data:
3, 8, 5, 8, 9, 10

8 occurs most often.

The mode is 8.

✎ Pencil Problem #3✎

3a. Find the mode for the following data:
7, 4, 3, 2, 8, 5, 1, 3

3b. Find the mode for the following data:
3, 8, 5, 8, 9, 3

Both 3 and 8 occur most often.

The modes are 3 and 8.

3b. Find the mode for the following data:
1.6, 3.8, 5.0, 2.7, 4.2, 4.2, 3.2, 4.7, 3.6, 2.5, 2.5

Copyright © 2017 Pearson Education, Inc.

3c. Find the mode for the following data:
3, 8, 5, 6, 9, 10

3c. Find the mode for the following data:
60, 70, 80, 50, 40, 30

Each data item occurs the same number of times.

There is no mode.

Answers for Pencil Problems *(Textbook Exercise references in parentheses)*:

1. 95 *(Appendix #3)*

2a. 60 *(Appendix #13)*   **2b.** 3.5 *(Appendix #9)*

3a. 3 *(Appendix #17)*   **3b.** 2.5 and 4.2 *(Appendix #23)*   **3c.** no mode *(Appendix #17-24)*

Homework:

☐ **Insert your homework** into this section of the *Learning Guide*. Show all work neatly and check your answers. Strive to work through difficulties when possible, making note of any exercises where you need additional help. Remember, even if your instructor assigns homework through *MyMathLab*, you should still write out your work.

Copyright © 2017 Pearson Education, Inc.